The Human Energy System

10/06

What is the human energy system? How does it function and what is our relationship to it? How does it affect our health, emotional and psychological well-being as well as our relationships? These are some of the thought provoking questions addressed in this book on healing.

Chakra Therapy is a practical and easy-to-use guide which describes the mechanics of the human energy systems and the dynamics of energy flow and energy interaction between you and others. This book will demonstrate that you are more than you think you are. You will learn that not only are you a physical being, you are a complex energy being who simultaneously communicates and receives nourishment from the physical plane, as well as the three subtle planes.

Here are exercises and techniques designed to increase your level of energy, to transmute unhealthy frequencies of energy into healthy ones, to bring you back into balance and harmony with your self, your loved ones, and the world you live in.

Human problems on all levels—spiritual, mental, emotional and physical—are caused by contraction, the inability to radiate energy freely due to blockages in the human energy system. You will learn how to release energy blockages, thereby healing yourself and enabling you to enjoy life to its fullest.

At this moment in history, the Earth and the human community, which includes every individual human being, suffers because of the poisoning of the physical environment. But the physical disease is merely the symptom of a deeper disease on the energy level. By healing ourselves energetically we begin to heal the collective energy field which surrounds us and permeates us and our planet. It is obvious that physical solutions no longer work and the planet cannot be healed by physical solutions alone. The hope of this generation lies within each person on the energy level. The time has come for a full understanding of ourselves and through this knowledge we receive the power to transform the multi-dimensional disease we all suffer from into the joy of perfect health.

About the Author

Keith Sherwood was born in New York in 1949. An internationally known teacher and healer, he founded the "American Psychic Association" and for two years was its director as well as editor of its magazine, *Psychic*. He has appeared on many radio and television shows in the United States and Europe. For three years he produced "Psychic Seminar," a weekly New York television program. He teaches "Chakra therapy," a synthesis of Western therapeutic techniques, Taoist Yoga and Tantra regularly throughout Europe.

His eclectic approach toward energy work is the outcome of years of study which took him first into psychotherapy as an encounter group therapist with New York City addicts. Later he traveled to the mountains of Guatemala where he studied with a Gurdieff master and trained in Yoga and Pranayama. He became a minister and worked in the Dominican Republic where his dormant powers as a healer and clairvoyant surfaced. After leaving the church in 1978 he devoted himself to the study of healing and human energy.

To Write to the Author

If you wish to contact the author or would like more information about this book, please write to the author in care of Llewellyn Worldwide, and we will forward you request. Both the author and publisher appreciate hearing from you and learning of your enjoyment of this book and how it has helped you. Llewellyn Worldwide cannot guarantee that every letter written to the author can be answered, but all will be forwarded. Please write to:

Keith Sherwood
c/o Llewellyn Worldwide
P.O. Box 64383-721, St. Paul, MN 55164-0383, U.S.A.

Please enclose a self-addressed, stamped envelope for reply, or $1.00 to cover costs.
If outside the U.S.A., enclose international postal reply coupon.

Free Catalog from Llewellyn

For more than 90 years Llewellyn has brought its readers knowledge in the fields of metaphysics and human potential. Learn about the newest books in spiritual guidance, natural healing, astrology, occult philosophy and more. Enjoy book reviews, new age articles, a calendar of events, plus current advertised products and services. To get your free copy of *Llewellyn's New Worlds of Mind and Spirit*, send your name and address to:

Llewellyn's New Worlds of Mind and Spirit
P.O. Box 64383-721, St. Paul, MN 55164-0383, U.S.A.

About Llewellyn's New Age Series

The "New Age"—it's a phrase we use, but what does it mean? Does it mean the changing of the Zodiacal Tides, that we are entering the Aquarian Age? Does it mean that a new Messiah is coming to correct all that is wrong and make Earth into a Garden? Probably not—but the idea of a *major change* is there, combined with awareness that Earth *can* be a Garden; that war, crime, poverty, disease, etc., are not necessary "evils."

Optimists, dreamers, scientists . . . nearly all of us believe in a "better tomorrow," but that somehow we can do things now that will make for a better future life for ourselves and for coming generations.

In one sense, we all know "there's nothing new under the Heavens," and in another sense that "every day makes a new world." The difference is in our consciousness. And this is what the New Age is all about: it's a major change in consciousness found within each of us as we learn to bring forth and manifest "powers" that Humanity has always potentially had.

Evolution moves in "leaps." Individuals struggle to develop talents and powers, and their efforts build a "power bank" in the Collective Unconsciousness, the "soul" of Humanity that suddenly makes these same talents and powers easier access for the majority.

Those who talk about a New Age believe a new level of consciousness is becoming accessible that will allow anyone to manifest powers previously restricted to the few who had worked strenuously for them: powers such as Healing (for self and others), Creative Visualization, Psychic Perception, Out-of-Body Consciousness and more.

You still have to learn the 'rules' for developing and applying these powers, but it is more like a "relearning" than a *new* learning, because with the New Age it is as if the basis for these had become genetic.

The books in the New Age series are as much about *Attitude* and *Awareness* as they are about the "mechanics" for learning and using Psychic, Mental, Spiritual, or Parapsychological Powers. Understanding that the Human Being is indeed a "potential god/goddess" is the first step toward the realization of that potential: expressing in outer life the inner creative powers.

Other Books by Keith Sherwood

Die Kunst Spirituellen Heilens
    (Hermann Bauer Verlag, West Germany, 1984)
The Art of Spiritual Healing
    (Llewellyn Publications, St. Paul, MN)

Forthcoming Titles:

The Inner World of Success

Llewellyn's New Age Series

CHAKRA THERAPY

For Personal Growth & Healing

Keith Sherwood

1996
Llewellyn Publications
St. Paul, Minnesota 55164-0383, U.S.A.

FIRST EDITION
Ninth Printing, 1996

Cover painting by Susan McDonnell
Illustrated by Jafus Trammell and Norman Stanley

Library of Congress Cataloging-in-Publication Data
Sherwood, Keith.
    Chakra therapy.

    (Llewellyn's new age series)
    1. Occultism. 2. Self—Miscellanea. 3. Chakras.
I. Title. II. Series.
BF1999.S46   1988   131   88-45186
ISBN 0-87542-721-9

Llewellyn Publications
A Division of Llewellyn Worldwide, Ltd.
P.O. 64383, St. Paul, MN 55164-0383

I would like to thank my teachers and students whose help was indispensable in the preparation of this book.

Contents

CHAPTER I

THE PSYCHOLOGY OF THE HUMAN ENERGY SYSTEM

Der Zweck des Lebens ist das Leben selbst.
(The aim of living is life itself)

—Goethe

Introduction

The study of human psychology and the study of humans themselves is incomplete without taking into consideration the human energy system and its profound effect on the human psyche, human behavior and human relationships. If a psychology of humans is to be truly useful and practical, it must describe a human as a total being, and it must provide the student with an understanding of a human in relationship to the world he/she lives in and the other beings he/she comes in contact with. A partial description like a piece of a pirates' map is practically useless, because it will not help a person find the treasure which he/she seeks. In human psychology, the treasure has always been happiness, a life which is balanced, harmonious and which allows room for love, trusting relationships and the experience of unconditional joy. We all want the map of human consciousness to lead us as quickly and efficiently as possible to the

1

treasure which we all intuitively know lives within us.

Unfortunately for most people, even with all the information available today they still haven't found their way home to them *selves*. They still don't know why they feel good one day, bad the next, why one morning they wake up full of energy, another morning they are more exhausted than when they went to bed. They don't know why they sometimes attract people and other times alienate them. In the midst of all their feelings, thoughts, ups and downs, the one thing they don't experience is consistency, wholeness and contentment, and they don't understand why. Despite the importance attached today to emotions, relationships and self-awareness, there remains an incredible lack of understanding and confusion about who we are and why we feel, think and act the way we do.

For more than 20 years I have studied human beings and the human energy system, and I have found that at the root of human problems are *energy problems*. Thoughts, feelings and actions are energy events. To know who you are and why you act, feel and think the way you do, you must know yourself *energetically*. You must realize how you influence others and how you are being influenced by energy—both your own energy, other people's energy, and the energy field which permeates and connects everything in the universe.

What You Will Learn

This book is meant first to fill in the missing pieces of a human's subtle anatomy left out by orthodox psychological models, then it will serve as a workbook. Within its pages are exercises and techniques designed to increase your level of energy, to transmute unhealthy frequencies of energy into healthy ones, to bring you back into balance and harmony with your self, your loved ones and the multidimensional world you live in. Finally, it will help bring you back into union with the universal field of energy and consciousness.

Human problems on all levels of causation—spiritual, mental, emotional and physical—are caused by contraction, the inability to radiate energy freely due to blockages in the human energy system. In this book you will learn how to release energy blockages and the reservoirs of energy these blockages create. These reservoirs of energy are the emotional and mental debris you weren't able to completely process through your energy system when you were a child. They are the result of energy overload, too much pain, fear, or anger caused by feelings which were too threatening, and shocks which were too powerful.

Once you have mastered the techniques presented here, you will have the capacity to release blockages and to transmute the reservoirs of energy which have been trapped by the blockages. With practice you will be able to change unhealthy frequencies of energy trapped by these blockages into healthy ones. Once you are able to transmute energy, you will have more energy in healthier frequencies at your disposal.

In this book you will also learn about *prana* which in Sanskrit means "absolute energy." Prana comes in many forms; sometimes it is called Ki, Chi, or Kundalini. You will study most intensively those frequencies which make up the human energy field and which influence human consciousness, human relationships and physical health. You will learn how Prana moves through your subtle energy system; the energy system composed of the chakras (energy transformers), the auras (energy reservoirs), and the nadis (energy channels), and how Prana interacts with the nervous system and the physical body. You will learn how Prana is transferred from one person to another, and how it can be absorbed and trapped in subtle and physical matter. You will learn about the various rays of Prana which human beings can and do project to each other, and you will learn how these rays influence human relationships.

Most importantly, you will learn how to heal yourself by healing your energy system. It is energy which is at the root of this study, because it is energy in its myriad forms which determines a person's physical health, emotional health, mental health and level of consciousness.

You Are an Energy Being

Before beginning, it is important for you to recognize that every living being is far more than just a physical being. Every living being is also an energy being. Each individual is composed of a system of energy fields which interact with each other and the environment they interpenetrate. The universe is permeated by these fields and a human being can be thought of as a localization or concentration in the universal field. The Taoists call this field the Tao. The Buddhists call it Brahma. Local fields not only interact with the universal field, but they interact with each other. Each thought, emotion and action can be viewed as an energy discharge radiating from a localized field, i.e. a person's personal energy field. The focal point from which energy radiates into the universal field we experience as "self." Our personal energy field "self" as well as everyone else's personal energy field resides and receives nourishment from the universal field. That is why on the inner levels we all are connected to one another.

It is written in the Bhagavad Gita "In abiding always in the eternal, the saint enjoys without effort the bliss which flows from realization of the infinite. He who experiences the unity of life sees his own self in all beings and all beings in his own self, and looks on everything with an impartial eye."[1]

It is because we all grow out of and are nourished from the same universal energy field, the same reservoir of Prana and consciousness, that makes it impossible to fully know ourselves unless we understand ourselves as energy beings, as part of the universal energy field. We distort reality if we think of ourselves as separate from everyone else and we distort reality if we think of our universe as limited to three dimensions.

We wear like a coat our consciousness (conscious mind) and the physical body and its senses which gather information about the physical world. It is necessary for our journey in physical reality to be conscious and to be wrapped in a physical body. But if a person identifies with their physical body, conscious mind and senses alone, believing that they are nothing more, they will not perceive the universe as it really is or experience their true relationship to it. By distorting reality and their experience of it, a person will disrupt their relationship to the universal field and all local fields within the universal field, including their own. Since we all have physical bodies and we are all conscious, it appears sensually that we are separate beings. But this is how it appears sensually only. The senses are only sensitive to a small part of the universal energy field, and even there they have their limitations. The truth is, we are interconnected and part of the same essential unity. We are localizations within the universal field of energy and consciousness.

Sub-Fields

In the same way that the physical body is composed of systems of interrelated organs, a person's personal energy field is composed of sub-fields which are interrelated and affect each other. These sub-fields are regulated by the organs of the subtle energy system, in particular the energy centers called chakras.

When any of the chakras or organs of the subtle energy system are disrupted or damaged, a particular sub-field is disrupted, energy becomes blocked, its frequency is distorted and the sub-field contracts. These blockages and disturbances are transmuted to neighboring sub-fields affecting them negatively and causing them to contract as well. These disruptions are the root cause of all forms of mental, emotional and physical disorders. It is these energy blockages which prevent a person from fully radiating energy and from experiencing him/herself as a complete, whole being.

Disturbances in the subtle energy system prevent a person from experiencing other people fully. They prevent a person from having intimate, completely satisfying relationships. Finally, disruptions and blockages in a person's sub-fields prevent a person from experiencing their natural state of union with the rest of the universal field.

Psycho-Spiritual Integration

The process of energy work which systematically changes unhealthy conditions in the human energy system and the human energy field into healthy ones I call *psycho-spiritual integration*. It is a system which promotes harmony and balance in the human energy field and the organs of the subtle energy system. It is a process which leads a person into a state of wholeness. Wholeness is achieved through self-remembrance, re-collection and re-union. Through self-remembrance, re-collection and re-union, a person comes back into direct experience of them *selves* as a complete, whole human being. They become in the end what I call the "I AM," the union of all "selves." In this state a person becomes fully conscious and is able to radiate energy fully from all his centers of power and consciousness.

By breaking energy blockages and releasing energy trapped in the subtle central energy system, an individual recovers, feels and consciously re-experiences old parts of self again. This is remembrance, and recollection of the lost parts follows. Recollection can be likened to collecting the parts together after they have been scattered. Reunion is the creative process whereby all the pieces are put together to form a whole. Reunion is the result of remembrance and recollection. Reunion leads to psychospiritual integration and the experience of the I AM as self. The I AM is the complete person. It is first experienced as a separate persona which resides deep within the unconscious. That is how it is experienced by an individual who has begun to remember who he/she is and to recollect the unconscious parts of him/herself together. To someone who has recollected all their unconscious selves, the I AM is experienced as the union of unconscious selves. An integrated person sees the I AM for what it truly is: the complete person with all selves, unconscious as well as conscious, in union with one another.

By breaking energy blockages, opening and balancing the chakras, facilitating remembrance, recollection and reunion, psycho-spiritual integration helps to bring a person back to his/her natural condition of wholeness. Once integration is achieved, a person will begin to experience him/herself as a whole being, in union with the rest of creation and as a result, they will again experience unconditional joy which is their birthright, the childlike state that Jesus spoke of when he said, "Verily I say unto you, except ye be converted and become as little children, ye shall not enter into the Kingdom of Heaven."[2]

The Second Attention

The I AM, the union of selves, experiences the universe differently from the conscious self which so many people identify as themselves. The I AM experiences the world subjectively by sensing energy fields. When something is experienced by the I AM, it is not only experienced for what it is but also for how it affects the feelings, thoughts and consciousness of the observer. The experience is not of qualities alone, but of a network of relationships, polarity, gender, cause and effect, rhythm and vibration, etc. In the I AM's relationship to the world, life exists everywhere in animate as well as inanimate matter on all levels of awareness. Everything breathes, everything pulses with life. There is a spirit in everything, and it is through this spirit (energy field) that the I AM makes contact and comes into relationship with everything in the manifest universe.

In order for the I AM to experience relationship with someone or something, a person must first develop the ability to sense the energy radiating from what they are experiencing in the form of fields and rays. A person does this by developing the second attention.

As human beings we experience the world in two ways. The first is through the five senses. Information from the physical environment, which includes the physical body, is experienced through one or more of the senses, is processed through the nervous system and interpreted by the rational mind. The interpretation is normally filtered through a reservoir of past experiences and knowledge. I call this the first attention and its main organs of cognition are the senses and the rational, analytical mind which are functions of consciousness. Its view of the universe is "me" centered and mechanical. Its cosmology is based ultimately on what ensures physical well-being and survival.

The second attention, however, is the attention of the I AM which experiences the world intuitively through the heart. Rather than being processed by the nervous system, the information received is processed by the subtle energy system (the chakras, auras, nadis) which experiences the world energetically by sensing energy fields. Energy fields are interdimensional and therefore not limited by space or time. Instead of basing its interpenetration on past experience, the second attention experiences the universe directly.

The first attention sees everything in the context of cause and effect. It sees itself in a three-dimensional universe held together by sequential time. The first attention sees the universe as orderly and predictable, as a great machine which runs according to rational mathematical rules. It predicts the future by knowing the present and remembering the past.

On the other hand, the second attention experiences the universe as an indivisible, dynamic whole, consisting of many dimensions, which interpenetrate one another, which are not subject to sequential time, and which can only be defined within the context of constantly shifting relationships. The second attention demands full participation which means *feeling*, sensing and touching the world, letting the world reach into it and allowing the world to make a deep impact on it at every moment.

The common expression of "being touched by an experience" will give you a good idea of what I mean. Developing the second attention means developing the ability to be affected, moved and permeated by experiences so that you participate with them fully on every level of causation. We can understand the second attention most easily if we use the analogy of a hologram. While the process of separation and observation is at the heart of the first attention, the second attention begins with the perception of unbroken wholeness. Like a hologram, its universe is " . . . implicate or enfolded . . . this means that each part, in some sense, contains the whole. If any part of the hologram is illuminated, the entire image will be reconstructed."[3] In the same way, the second attention sees the whole in each piece and each piece in the whole. The second attention perceives the world intuitively and perceives "mind and matter as being interdependent and correlated . . . They are mutually enfolding projections of a higher reality . . . "[4]

The second attention is the innate capacity each of us has to perceive our inner and outer environment intuitively through the heart and unconscious mind. We can think of it as a window through which the I AM sees and experiences the manifest world. By developing the second attention by cleaning the window and keeping it free from obstructions, the I AM will have a clear view of what is taking place. Developing the second attention and keeping the window free of obstructions so that the I AM can emerge is essential in the work of psychospiritual integration.

CHAPTER II

DEVELOPING THE SECOND ATTENTION

> Warriors prepare themselves to be aware, and
> full awareness comes to them only when there is
> no more self-importance left in them.
> —Carlos Castaneda
> *The Fire From Within*

In this chapter you will learn, through a week-long series of
exercises, a method for developing the "second attention,"
the attention of the I AM as it experiences the world intuitively through the heart. Developing the second attention
begins when you become "detached" from your actions,
mentally, emotionally and physically and you begin observing what you do. This is called *checking*.

In the series of exercises presented below you will
learn first how to check yourself, then you will learn to
experience the world through the second attention. Like a
doctor, in checking you must be cool and objective, you
must stand outside the activity you are doing. In all the
exercises in this chapter, you will do your checking on three
levels: physical, emotional and mental. On Day One you
will be using a recent photograph of yourself, which you
will also use on Day Three. You will also be using a photo
of yourself as an adolescent, and lastly a photo of yourself

as a child, both of which you will use on Day Four. Before you begin the first exercise, choose the photos you plan to use. They should be full length pictures, preferably of you alone.

Day One

Begin by sitting in a comfortable position and study the most recent picture of yourself. Start on the physical level by checking for areas of stiffness or tension, areas where you seem tight and might be storing pain, fear or anger. Ask yourself questions (I suggest you write out your questions and jot down the answers that come to you so that you can review them later). Ask yourself if this person looks relaxed or does he or she look tense, are they carrying themself naturally or do their movements or positions suggest they are hiding something? Be specific and make note of all areas that do not seem to be open and relaxed. On the emotional level, pay attention to what the person in the photograph is feeling. Are they happy or sad, content or discontent? What feelings are they expressing? Ask yourself if this person is expressing them inappropriately? Then ask yourself, do you like the expression on this person's face? If you do, fine, but if you don't, ask yourself why not.

Finally, move to the mental level and while studying the picture, try to experience what the person in the picture is experiencing mentally. Let their thoughts become your thoughts. Ask yourself if you looked like them what would you be thinking, or would you be thinking at all? Perhaps your mind would be perfectly clear. If not, put words to the person's thoughts and for a few moments think the same thoughts they are thinking. After you have studied the photo for a few minutes and you have written down the questions and answers for later study, study the photos of yourself as an adolescent and a child in the same manner.

After you are finished, lie down on a flat surface with

your hands comfortably at your sides. Continue the exercise by checking yourself in your present condition—physically, emotionally, and mentally. Then begin breathing deeply through your nose in a relaxed and regular rhythm. When you feel ready, bring your attention to your feet; draw in your breath and contract the muscles of your feet as much as possible. Hold your breath for three seconds. After three seconds, release your breath and allow the muscles of your feet to relax. Inhale deeply again and repeat the procedure, this time with your ankles and calves. Continue by repeating the same procedure with the following parts of your body: your thighs, your buttocks, neck, arms and then the hands. Next, squeeze the muscles of your face and hold for three seconds. After three seconds, release and exhale. Now open your mouth, stick out your tongue and stretch the muscles of your face as much as possible; hold your breath for three seconds, then release the muscles of your face and exhale.

To complete this part of the exercise, contract your entire body (this time squeezing the muscles of your face), and hold your breath. Finally, after three seconds expel the air forcibly through your nose while releasing all the muscles of your body at once. Then pay attention to your physical body and "check" how it feels. Pay attention to the subtle vibrations and energies which are flowing through it. Check for areas of tension or tightness. Check for areas which feel numb, which seem to have a lack of feeling. Then pay attention to your emotions, watch them as they flow through you but don't get attached to any of them; simply check them. Ask yourself: what am I feeling, where are these feelings centered? Am I resisting them or letting them flow through me? Have I judged them and if I have, what is my judgement? Finally, check your mind by paying attention to the spontaneous images flowing through it. Stay detached from your thoughts. Make no attempt to control them; simply watch them. Continue to be the observer and watch yourself without making any attempt to modify or change your condition physically, emotionally or mentally. Continue checking yourself on all levels for about ten minutes or until you feel satisfied, then open your eyes. You will feel wide awake, perfectly relaxed and better than you did before.

Day Two

Repeat the tensing and releasing exercise from Day One, except that after you have completed it, instead of observing your condition, visualize and experience yourself getting up and walking ten steps away from your body. It is important that you keep all your senses open and alert so that besides seeing yourself walking ten steps beyond your body, you experience the action physically, emotionally and mentally. After you have taken ten steps, turn around slowly, walk back and lie down again in your body. Remember, even though it is important to experience yourself walking away and returning as fully as possible, remain an observer. Don't get attached to what you are doing. Just keep checking the person who is walking physically, emotionally and mentally. After you have lain back inside yourself, relax for about 10 minutes and when you are satisfied, open your eyes. You will feel wide awake, perfectly relaxed and better than you did before.

Day Three

For the exercise on Day Three you will need the recent photo of yourself that you have chosen. I recommend that you do this exercise in a sitting position. The photo should stand in front of you so that you can see it clearly without moving your head. Once you have set the photo in front of you, close your eyes and begin breathing deeply and rhythmically through your nose until you feel relaxed.

Then bring your attention to your toes. If you pay attention to them for even a few moments you will feel them tingle. You will feel a vibration in your toes caused by circulation. Feel the vibration spread through your feet and feel your feet relax. Continue this part of the exercise by paying attention to your ankles. Pay attention to them until they begin to tingle and relax. You might find it helpful to visualize yourself massaging and stroking your ankles. You can use this visualization for any part of your body you think it will benefit.

Continue the process of physical relaxation by bringing your attention to your calves. From there move to your knees. From your knees feel the tingling sensation move to your thighs. Pay attention to your thighs until they are completely relaxed. Continue in this way with your hips, your buttocks, pelvic region, lower abdomen and lower back, upper abdomen and middle back. Then feel the tingling sensation in your chest and shoulders. After you feel your shoulders relax, focus your attention on your fingers. Continue the process of relaxation with your fingers, hands, wrists, lower arms, elbows, upper arms; then move to your neck and throat. Your face gets special attention. Most people have emotional tensions stored in the muscles of their face. Start with your jaw, then go to your chin, mouth, cheeks, nose, ears, eyes, forehead; feel the tingling sensation move up the back of your neck, and finally feel your entire scalp tingling and relaxing completely. After you have become completely conscious of your body, open your eyes, but not completely. Keep them slightly unfocused and look at the picture in front of you. Repeat the exercise that you just completed with the person in the photo. Begin with their toes and check for the vibration. Then go to their feet and finally go through their whole body feeling the vibration in each part of their body and feeling each part of their body relaxing. After you have finished, close your eyes and relax for about ten minutes. When you feel satisfied, open your eyes again. You will feel wide awake, perfectly relaxed and better than you did before.

Day Four

You begin the exercise on Day Four in a sitting position with the recent photo in front of you just like on Day Three. Begin by closing your eyes and breathing rhythmically through your nose until you feel relaxed. Next open your eyes for a moment, keep them slightly unfocused and look at the picture in front of you for a count of three. Then immediately close your eyes and mentally visualize what you saw in the picture for 20 seconds. Repeat the procedure two more times. After the third repetition, open your eyes and look at the photo again, but this time pay particular attention to emotions the person in the photo is expressing. Close your eyes again for 20 seconds more and visualize the photo again, but this time go one step further. Empathize with the person in the photo and check them emotionally so that you *feel* their feelings. Repeat your checking two more times in the same way. After the third repetition, open your eyes, look at the photo and let yourself experience the mental state that is expressed by the person in the photo. After a count of three, close your eyes, then visualize and experience the mental state that is expressed by the person in the photo. Repeat this two more times for 20 seconds each time. After the third repetition, close your eyes and relax for ten minutes. When you open your eyes you will feel wide awake, relaxed and better than you did before.

Day Five

On Day Five, repeat the same exercise you did on Day Four using the two other photos you chose earlier: one of yourself as an adolescent and one of yourself as a child.

Day Six

Begin the exercise on Day Six in a sitting position in front of a full length mirror; if you don't have a full length mirror, use the biggest one you have. Sit about six feet away from it. Go through the awareness exercise you did on Day Three. After you are finished, repeat the visualization exercise you did on Day Four, except that you substitute the image of yourself in the mirror for the photo. However, instead of doing the exercise for 20 seconds at a time, extend the duration to 40 seconds. When you are finished, relax for about ten minutes. Then open your eyes. When you do, you will feel wide awake, perfectly relaxed and better than you did before.

Day Seven

On the seventh day you will put together everything you learned from the previous six days. Begin by finding a comfortable sitting position. Close your eyes and breathe deeply and rhythmically through your nose until you feel relaxed. Sit quietly, breathing in this way for about ten minutes. Then do the awareness exercise you learned on Day Three. After you finish the awareness exercise, check yourself. Check yourself physically, emotionally and mentally. Stay detached. Watch yourself objectively in the same way a critic watches an actor perform his part in the theater. Then let the actor get up and go for a walk. This is an actual walk, not a visualization. Empathize with the actor so that you experience what the actor feels physically, emotionally and mentally as he is walking. Walk for about 20 minutes in this state of consciousness, and keep checking the actor. When you return to your seat 20 minutes later, relax for about five minutes in your ordinary state of consciousness with your eyes closed, breathing deeply and rhythmically through your nose. When you open your eyes, you will feel wide awake, perfectly relaxed and better than you did before.

If you were successful in checking and staying detached during your walk, you will now know what I am talking about when I speak of the second attention. It is a very different state of consciousness and a very different way of perceiving the world. It is one you must develop and use, because without it you will be unable to experience the world fully enough to achieve a continual state of unconditional joy which is the goal of psychospiritual integration. If you were not completely successful in this week-long program, repeat the program again for another week and do the exercises twice daily. If after a second week you are not completely successful, repeat the program again. Repeat it for as long as necessary in order to achieve a working knowledge of the second attention. It is through the second attention that the I AM makes contact and comes into relationship with everything in the manifest universe. It is through the second attention that the I AM experiences its connection to the universal energy field and the personal fields within it.

As Jung said:

> . . . we become conscious of ourselves through self-knowledge and . . . In this way there arises a consciousness which is no longer imprisoned in the petty, oversensitive personal world of the ego, but participates freely in the wider world of objective interests. This widened consciousness is no longer that touchy, egotistical bundle of personal wishes, fears, hopes and ambitions which has always to be compensated or corrected by unconscious counter-tendencies, instead it is a function of relationship to the world of objects, bringing the individual into absolute binding and indissoluble communion with the world at large.

CHAPTER III

ORIGINAL SEPARATION

What one could almost call a systematic blindness is simply the effect of the prejudice that God is outside man.

—C. G. Jung
The Illness That We Are

The notion that humans are incomplete and that they can become separated from the universal field is held as an objective reality in the Judeo-Christian world. The views of psycho-spiritual integration are at odds with this notion.

The techniques of psycho-spiritual integration are designed to shatter the false sense of separation which prevents a person from consciously experiencing their unity with the universal field, and participating in the unconditional joy of union with it.

The striking difference between orthodox Christianity, Judaism, and psycho-spiritual integration is that both the Christian and the Jew believe that a human is born in a separate condition (original sin) and that even after conversion he/she can separate him/herself from the universal field of energy and consciousness through sin, and that in this condition a person is spiritually dead. In integration we don't accept a person's original state as one of separation, and we don't accept separation as objectively the truth. Although a person might not experience their inner life consciously and might do those things which constantly push them further from an experience of it, it remains that on the unconscious level they have never been separate and can never be separate from the universal field. S/he exists within the universal field whether they believe it or not, or whether they consciously experience it or not. S/he has always been and always will be in the Tao, Brahma, what Christians call the "mind of Christ." Moreover, on the unconscious level they continually experience, communicate, and receive nourishment from the universal field.

Each person exists within this field and receives the benefits of it just like Jesus or any enlightened master. The only difference is that the enlightened master experiences his union with the universal field consciously as well as unconsciously. He has freed himself from the illusion that only what exists in the physical world is real. He understands who he is in relationship to the universal energy field and the consciousness which pervades it, because he directly experiences the universal field and the "All," the universal consciousness which supports the field. He is able to experience the universal field consciously by resisting the tendency to identify with his conscious mind and physical senses to the exclusion of everything else. Instead, by putting all the parts of himself together, he melts into the "I AM" which is a synthesis of "selves," and through the I AM he experiences himself in proper relationship to the "All" and everything else contained within the "All."

Judeo-Christian Tradition

The foundation of Western thought was laid down by Judaic scholars and theologians. In the Judaic tradition we have the notion that the Hebrew people are chosen by God but have become separated from Him and the notion that the Jewish people are inherently different from their brothers, inherently separate. At the heart of these notions is the institutionalization of separation. The Hebrew predicament was how to please a jealous and demanding God. In the books of Isaiah, the prophet rebukes the children of Israel. He tells them "your iniquities have separated you and your God and your sins have hid His face from you, that He will not hear."[1] Again in Leviticus God speaks through the prophet and says: "But I have said unto you, Ye shall inherit their land, and I will give it unto you to possess it, a land that floweth with milk and honey; I am the lord your God, which have separated you from other people."[2]

Although Jesus came preaching that each person was inherently like Him and that they had direct access to the Father (the universal field of energy and consciousness) by surrendering to Him through the person of the Holy Spirit, Christian theology became rigid and dogmatic, emphasizing the form rather than the spirit of Jesus' teaching. Like the Pharisees before them, in part because they embraced Aristotelian thought, Christian theologians now preach that man is at birth a divided being. The Apostle Paul tells us in the book of Galations: "Walk in the spirit and ye shall not fulfill the lust of the flesh. For the flesh lusteth against the Spirit, and the Spirit against the flesh: and these are contrary one to the other."[3] This verse as well as many others have been used by clergymen throughout the centuries to support the notion that man stands outside the universal field, that he lives in a state of separation where everything is either I, Me or the "other." From Christian doctrine we learn that man in his primordial state (in the Garden of Eden) experienced life without duality, he experienced it in its unity through his connection with God. But through sin (which in Greek means separation) man became fragmented and lost his experience of unity. For the Christian, Jesus became the advocate, who intercedes with the Father on fallen humanity's behalf and as a result, He becomes the bridge between spirit (the father) and flesh (humanity). Through Jesus who has now become Christ, the I AM, in His function as intercessor, humanity again has access to the Father, the "All" which was lost due to Adam's sin. Through Jesus man can become whole again by regaining access to the subtle worlds through Jesus' special relationship with the Father. As Jesus Himself tells His disciples " . . . and no man knoweth who the son is, but the Father; and who the Father is, but the son, and whom the son will reveal him."[4]

It is this access to the inner worlds, the Christian tells us, which was lost when Adam was forced out of the garden. For the Christian, Jesus is the archetype of man undivided, man in union with the universal field, the "All." Jesus became the Christ, the "Anointed One" by breaking through the illusion of Maya (fragmentation). By becoming whole He experienced the anointing of Prana which flows undisturbed to those who have broken through duality and have become the I AM.

Christ In You

But the important question for those brought up in a Christian world is: was Jesus fundamentally different from everyone else? There is no question that quantitatively He was different, if we are able to believe He performed the miracles the Gospels tell us He performed. But qualitatively, even He insisted there was no difference. He claimed that He was the first of many brothers.

Although they may grow up differently, brothers come from the same mother, in this case the universal field, and they are always in union with the universal field. As the Kenopanisad tells us " . . . all the parts of my body, my eyes, ears, speech and life, all the strength of my senses get nourishment (in Him). All beings are actually Brahma . . . "[5]

Duality

The doctrine of separation, which is at the root of orthodox theology and is the cause of so much misunderstanding and unnecessary suffering, is the foundation of orthodox psychology as well. Orthodox psychology built its towers on the shoulders of Newtonian and Cartesian thought which saw separation as the natural human condition. By building upon the Aristotelian model and by basing so much of its research and doctrine on empirical evidence, the Christian church and orthodox psychology have until now failed to see man in his completeness, as the multidimensional being he is. By building upon the tradition of Aristotle, Socrates and Plato, the Church saw man within the context of his "duality."

Plato saw man as continually striving between what was base in his nature and what was noble. Sitting between these conflicting elements was the element of soul called *Thymos* (the element of courage) which was the bridge between the noble aspiration of the mind and man's animal, carnal desires. The main trend in Platonic thought was the understanding of man's inherently dual nature. Aristotle expanded on Platonic thought, but he still saw man in his duality. Aristotle taught his students that by acting courageously, a man chooses to identify with what is noble in his character and to reject what is base. But this form of courage includes the inevitable repression of those elements in his nature which he considers ignoble. They are rejected, and rather than being integrated they are judged, sentenced and become the "others" within himself.* In the Aristotelian view it is what is praiseworthy which must triumph over what is not. This Aristotelian duality is carried over to

---

* The "others" are those unwanted, unloved parts of self which exist deep within the unconscious of an unintegrated person. They are the little demons which were first rejected by a parent and then by the child who rejected a part of themself to regain the loss of love and relationship with the parent. It is particularly these "others" within unconsciousness which must be remembered, recollected and reunited with each other and the conscious self.

Christian thought and into rationalism which gave birth to modern science and psychology.

Newton and his contemporaries, the founders of modern Western science (in particular Descartes), firmly pushed the Western world into the bed of rationalism and materialism. Rationalism and materialism triumphed over a medieval world which, although laboring under a theology based on duality, still had its roots deeply imbedded in intuition and faith. Moreover, in the medieval world God was still at the center of the universe, and the overwhelmingly agrarian society of the day still had its roots extending back to our earliest ancestors, who saw life in everything and reality as often subjective. To medieval man, everything besides man himself was still a reflection of God (and was still in union with the universal field of energy and consciousness). But with Newton, Descartes and their contemporaries who ushered in the scientific revolution, God was pushed out of the center of the solar system. The whole became fragmented, what was organic became mechanical. The universe became a great machine, which God had set in motion and then left.

Descartes made scientific thought analytical and subject to pure reasoning. He pursued his work by dividing nature into manageable pieces and analyzing each piece thoroughly in order to understand its true nature. Of course, in this mechanical universe there was no room for unity, for a universal field, a spirit, or even a possibility for an overall governing purpose or intent at the root of the phenomenal universe. Nor could there be anything outside a universe that could not be weighed or measured.

Everything outside physical reality was hallucination or simply flights of fancy, the products of an unruly or primitive mind.

The science of Descartes, Newton and their contemporaries divided the world into parts, refusing to see it ecologically, to see it as a unified field. As time passed, the outer fragmentation led to inner fragmentation. It led to a shattering of man's concept of himself existing within the field of an omnipresent God. Man became a separate mechanical being, a machine living in a universe filled with other machines, who could be studied outside the context of his environment. His spiritual nature was ignored and his inner realities ridiculed. Man, like his universe, became fragmented; he became divided against himself.

Freud and many of his contemporaries accepted man divided. They saw him as an id, ego and superego, each striving continually against the other. Moreover, in their theories which were the final triumph of reason over intuition, duality over unity, they cut man off from his spiritual source of nourishment which is the universal field of energy and consciousness, and thus Nietzsche's bold statement "God is dead," and Marx' indictments against religion triumphed over thousands of years of experience and intuitive knowledge which taught that man no longer connected to a universal energy field and consciousness becomes a machine, albeit an extraordinary machine, but finite, mortal and ultimately alone with no access to higher planes. Freud saw man's need to experience higher consciousness and to achieve integration as an infantile need to return to the womb. By not seeing it as the profound yearning for wholeness and self-realization, Freud condemned man to an incomplete experience of himself.

As reason triumphed over intuition, man's inner life drowned under the weight of cold analytical reason and logic. Coming from this philosophical base, neither the modern Christian Church or orthodox psychology has been able to offer man a way home to himself, to a place of rest. Rather they have settled for tranquilizing people and filling them with false hope, so that they become numbed to the fear and pain, which gnaws at them in the depths of their being.

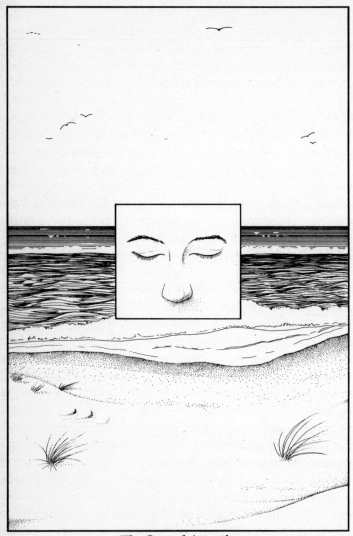

The Second Attention

Use the Second Attention as a window to view the world with accuracy.

CHAPTER IV

THE ROOT OF YOUR PROBLEM

... In the depths, down I must bore. There is
peace for eternity.

—Henrik Ibsen
The Miner

Although objectively every person is in union with the
universal field, the conscious experience of union has been
disrupted for most people by a disruption in their personal
energy field. When a person's personal energy field is disrupted persistently over a long period of time, they will
forget their original state of union which they experienced
as an infant and consciously they will experience only
separation and the existential pain which accompanies it.
Unfortunately, this has become the condition of the vast
majority of people. Most people today are still unaware that
at the root of every human problem is an energy problem.
They are unaware that to solve problems and achieve life
goals, they must change the quantity and quality of energy
flowing through their subtle energy system, and they must
change their relationship to the energy field which surrounds and permeates them.

I wrote this book because in the years I have studied
and become proficient in the use and transmutation of

energy, I have marveled at the lack of understanding and the inability people have in working with energy. Most people fail in their efforts to improve and develop themselves because they don't understand that the cause of their problems are disruptions in their subtle energy system and personal energy field. Even if they *do* make this cognitive breakthrough, they rarely have the tools they need to repair prior damage to their energy system.

My Life Didn't Work

I have devoted the greater part of my life to energy work, not initially for any altruistic purpose . . . very few people begin the work of psycho-spiritual integration for the right reasons; but because like many people, my life simply didn't work. By the time I reached adolescence I was spending the greater part of my time trying to figure out what was wrong with my life rather than living it. This caused me all sorts of suffering because I sought to pin myself down, to know myself by knowing the different parts of myself. I mistakenly believed that in this way I could know who I was and what I should do with my life.

I later learned that my problem was not that I did not know who I was, the problem was that I put that question to myself in the first place. The question, "Who am I?" can never be answered, and all it leads to is striving, pushing and pulling, further separation and inner turmoil. As I learned later, I asked the question in order to avoid the pain of experiencing the "others" within me . . . the little demons lurking in my unconscious. The avoidance of "these others," rather than easing my suffering actually caused me more suffering. There came a time when the suffering became so pervasive that I could not remember an earlier time when I was free from it.

The attempt to know myself, to resolve my inner conflict, to ease my suffering and to achieve some semblance of peace and harmony led me inexorably into the study of my subtle energy system. I learned the principles of psycho-spiritual integration a little at a time, and as I did, I remembered and re-collected hitherto lost and unwanted parts of myself. As I began to recollect "the others" buried within me, my life became more joyful and began to work better. I developed me and released the energy imprisoned within. I developed the system I present to you here, the system I call psycho-spiritual integration, out of necessity, out of my need to understand and integrate the seemingly contradictory parts of myself.

Growing Up

Because I was sensitive as a child, not only did I suffer from fragmentation but I was bombarded by the energy radiating from the energy fields of other people in the form of thoughts, feelings and bodily sensations without being aware of it. If I was around someone whose mind was full of negative thoughts, my mind would absorb them. If the person projected negative emotions, I absorbed them as well. I even picked up headaches and other minor pains and ailments from other people without realizing it.

When I reached adolescence, difficulties at home and at school plus the lack of understanding and support which accompanied sexual maturity all contributed to the crisis which brought me face to face with myself and the conflicting desires, feelings and ideas which were the baggage I had accumulated from early childhood. It was within the context of my adolescent crisis that I made the decision to find answers to my problems by looking within myself. My crisis was not unique and it does not make me different from anyone else. We all face this crisis in one degree or another. It is merely a person's relationship to the crisis and to its resolution which determines the direction a person takes, whether they will actively seek psycho-spiritual integration or whether they will accept life and themselves as fragmented.

The difference between my life and so many others is that I actively and consciously sought to understand what was blocking me and to remove the blockages so that I could experience life in its fullness. I emerged from my adolescent crisis with one goal which became my passion: to be completely myself, to radiate freely without fear, no matter what the circumstances. From that time, experiencing myself and being myself became my life's work.

Studying Everyone Else

As I progressed, I learned that by studying myself I was also studying everyone else, because regardless of where we live or from what culture we come, on an energy level we are all the same—we are, as it were, all made by the same manufacturer. With each new bit of understanding I came closer to my goal, closer to experiencing the essential unity which underlies everything. William James tells us, "Now in all of us, however constituted, but to a degree the greater in proportion as we are intense and sensitive and subject to diversified temptations . . . does the normal evolution of character chiefly consist in the straightening out and unifying of the inner self. The higher and lower feeling, the useful and true erring impulses, begin by being a comparative chaos within us—they must end by forming a stable system of functions in right subordination. Unhappiness is apt to characterize the period of order-making and struggle."[1]

James goes on by giving us the example of St. Augustine whose inner crisis is well-known and documented in Augustine's biography. James tells us, "Saint Augustine's psychological genius has given an account of the trouble of having a divided self which has never been surpassed."[2] In his biography, Augustine explains subsequent to his conversion to Christianity, "The new will which I began to have was not yet strong enough to overcome that other will, strengthened by long indulgence. So these two wills, one old, one new, one carnal, the other spiritual, contended with each other and disturbed my soul."³

Like Augustine, the fragmented parts of myself centered with each other, and as a result I had no sudden revelation of conversion which brought me back to a state of unconditional joy. I had to remember, recollect and reunite the buried scattered parts of my "self." The idea of one catharsis changing a person's life completely and ultimately is unrealistic. Change is gradual. A sudden spontaneous change only appears spontaneous to our conscious self, but in our unconscious there are usually months of unseen preparatory work.

Dr. Robert Assagioli speaks of a period of "psychic gestation," a period in which the unconscious mind assimilates experiences. Our conscious experiences stimulate latent forces already present within our unconscious, within our higher bodies, but the unconscious needs time for processing these experiences and for blockages to loosen. This process is rhythmic, with times of gestation and then times of sudden spontaneous transformation. I had hundreds of revelations and conversions all of which helped me remember, recollect and reunite the lost parts of my self. The crisis I experienced in my youth pushed me first into a series of cathartic experiences, but later these experiences became so ubiquitous in my life that they became process, and the process in time brought me face to face with the union of selves, the I AM.

Personal Responsibility

For me the road back began in earnest when I stopped blaming everyone else for my miserable condition and started to take responsibility for my own state of being. As soon as I accepted the fact that I had chosen to contract, I realized that I could choose to radiate again. So I began looking for a handle, something I could get hold of, which would bring me inside myself where some changes could be made. It seemed to me that if I could find some tools to release my blocked emotions, I could get back on the track and get on with my life. I began to explore. Fortunately I fell into a program which was pioneered by Daniel Caserall and Arthur Janov. It was a program of group encounters. The major tool of encounter group therapy as it was then called, was confrontation and the experience of "primals." When a group member was being dishonest, and I do not mean giving false information, but rather when he was falsifying his emotions, either blocking them or indulging in them, he was confronted and the group demanded that his real feelings be expressed. Moreover, behavior which institutionalized these inappropriate emotions or blocked inappropriate emotions from radiating freely was unacceptable to the group, and the group member was expected to change such behavior. He was expected to take the risk of changing those things in his life which prevented him from living and expressing himself honestly. Group members learned to release old fears, anger and pain which had been bottled up within them for years. Once the emotions were released it became easier to change old habits and to stop acting out old "stuff." It became easier to be honest and to relate more adult-like in the here and now.

Marathon

One group experience was particularly significant for me. It illustrates how energy in the form of emotions can be trapped within a person's personal energy field and can affect their lives for years. It took place during a marathon, an 18 hour group which lasted all night in Woodstock, New York in 1972. The group began about 6 p.m. For most of the night I was assisting the group leader Al. Around 2 a.m., just after some of us had eaten a snack, one group member began to speak. He spoke about not being good enough for his parents, about the fact that nothing he could do seemed to be enough to make them happy. He began to cry as he spoke. I could feel the sadness radiating from him. The feeling became contagious and it rapidly spread throughout the group. It struck a deep chord which seemed to run through almost everyone. It was the deep nagging feeling that no matter how much we worked or tried, we were not good enough for our parents and no matter how we tried, somehow there was something deep inside that was wrong, that doomed us and prevented us from getting what we needed to be happy and content. I couldn't help but empathize with the other group members and the hopeless feeling which had been buried deep within them. After a few moments I began to feel a heaviness on my chest. I hadn't felt it for a long time, but I remembered it right away. It was a feeling I dreaded, it was one I felt as a child, one I was frightened of, which I repressed and tried to avoid at all costs. It made me feel horrible. It sucked the joy out of everything. If I put words to it, it would say, "joy is fleeting, but I last forever. Nothing you do is enough, you'll never rid yourself of me." I could see that almost everyone else felt the same way I did. We were, for the first time since we began almost eight hours before, acknowledging the fact that we all were in the same boat, all in the same way deprived as children, all in our own way reaching out for love.

I began to feel sad as he spoke, sad because I saw that I was deeply wounded and so was everyone else in the group. In that very moment I wanted to reach out, I wanted to help the other group members, to comfort them in some way, to soothe their pain. Their pain highlighted mine and it forced me to acknowledge my own need for comfort. I could feel my own hurt, and in the moment of recognition I felt compassion for the little boy within me who was so confused and suffered for so long. I saw that everyone else had been deeply injured like I had been and I could feel tears of compassion coming to my eyes. I felt such a profound sadness that I felt I might break if someone didn't come quickly and hold me together. Other people were crying in different corners of the room and somehow the whole room changed complexion, as if a shade had come and softened everything.

For some reason I couldn't stand the exposure of sitting within the group, so I slipped out of my chair, stepped back a few steps and sat against the wall with my legs up— just letting myself relax, and somehow it was easier because I was more alone where I was. I closed my eyes and felt tired, and weary. I saw my parents in my mind and after so many years of blaming them for my unhappiness I didn't want to blame them anymore. I just wanted to rest. I could only think of how hurt their childhood must have been, and I felt sorry for them and wished that their parents had been able to care more for them. I could not blame them anymore for not understanding me and mistreating me. It seemed so mean and small when I thought of how difficult their lives must have been. For the first time (and this surprised me), I remembered my mother holding me in her arms; I remembered feeling safe then. I couldn't remember feeling that secure for years.

It must have been a while that these thoughts and feelings were going through me, because when I opened my eyes I saw that the chairs had been pushed aside and that almost everyone was sitting on the floor and that their attention was focused on me. Al was sitting on my right side. I was embarrassed and suprised and I looked away. "Oh lord," I whispered under my breath, and someone put their arm around my shoulder. I wanted to scream, "do not touch me, just leave me alone," but the words just wouldn't form in my throat and I squeezed my eyes together trying to fight off the inevitable release which was welling up inside of me.

I heard a voice say "Why don't you just give up Keith?" It was Al. He repeated it, "why don't you just give up? You can never be good enough for them, you could never be what they wanted you to be; just give up." I couldn't answer and I heard him say again "open your mouth and just say it, 'I give up'." I did what he told me.

At first my words were so soft, only I could hear them. But after a few moments the dam broke and the words came pouring out; the words "I give up."

Two other hands took hold of me and I heard other voices. Gently I was stretched out on the floor and within a few moments my hands and feet began to tingle and my head became so light I felt a little dizzy. Someone took my hand and from all around I felt love flowing through me. As I lay there repeating over and over again "I give up," I began to feel as if the burdens of the world which I had been carrying for so long were being lifted from my shoulders. At that moment of catharsis I reached beyond the pain and aloneness to a time when I was unconditionally loved and accepted. I could feel my mother's energy envelop me and interpenetrate me, becoming part of me, and it was in that moment that I realized that to reject my pain was to reject her and to reject her I must reject myself. I saw clearly for the first time that to have rejected her energy was to have rejected an essential part of my personal energy field. In the same way that we are physically the product of our mother and father, energetically we are also a product, a synthesis of our mother's and father's energy fields. As we grow older, we integrate other frequencies of energy into our personal energy field—but to reject or forget something as basic as the vibration of "mother" or "father" is to do terrible damage to one's energy system.

As I lay there I kept repeating softly, "I give up, I give up." The more I said it, the more a sense of peace enveloped me. There was nothing I could do—I couldn't change anything. All I could do was give up, forget that I had so many problems and just let things be. The feelings that enveloped me were so serene and peaceful, they seemed sacred as if I somehow was being bathed in a divine energy. My eyes were closed and I rested. There was no sense of time or place. There was only peace. I could feel Al's hand on my forehead; it ws a good feeling and it added to the profound sense of joy I was experiencing. I lay there for a long time and could feel after awhile that I should be alone.

Al whispered to me "Keith, stay with us and tell us what's happening."

"I have to be alone" was all I could answer. I walked across the room and felt that each person was part of me and I wanted to touch each one in some way, but I knew that I shouldn't, at least not then. So I left the house and stepped into the yard and began to walk slowly toward a stream which was nearby. I could hardly feel myself walking. I could only feel the elements which were touching me, the water which I seemed to hear with a greater intensity than ever before and the breeze I seemed to feel more deeply than ever before. Looking up into the early morning sky I could see millions of stars, and as I looked, I felt waves of energy flowing over me and the warmth was inexpressible. One after another, the waves of energy flowed over me and through me.

After awhile, everything inside of me began to liquify and then vaporize and I did not feel myself anymore. I just *felt*, and I knew I was crying like I had never cried before. I could see and feel lights radiating through me, and I felt grateful as I sat by the stream and watched and saw things which I had always taken for granted. I was at peace, and peace was somehow more than I ever imagined it could be, because it was electric. It pulsated and it breathed, and it wasn't at all quiet or dull. It made sitting the most exciting experience of my life.

CHAPTER V

CLIMBING THE MOUNTAIN

... It is not sufficient for us to enter into ourselves. It is not enough for us to realize that the spirituality of our nature makes us potentially God-like. The potentiality must be actualized by knowledge and love.

—Merton
The New Man

After two and one half years in group therapy, I became a therapist and worked in the city of New York with drug abusers leading encounter groups. While I worked as a therapist I began to study Yoga, Pranayama and meditation. I continued these studies until I met my teacher three years later. During the time I spent with him, I traveled extensively throughout North and Central America. The basic thrust of his teaching was that true knowledge (knowledge which was cathartic) came from the ALL directly through the unconscious. In order to bring us into direct relationship to the ALL, he taught us to pay attention and to remember who we were. He explained that a person must become "nobody" (childlike) again. Only from that position could a person be empty enough for the true self, the I AM, to emerge. When the true self emerged, it would express itself predominantly in two ways. It would express itself through clarity and thankfulness.

I remained with my teacher for three years. In the spring of 1975, we returned to New York after several months in Guatemala. It was when we arrived in New York that he told me he had taught me everything he could and that our relationship as student and teacher was over. "From now on," he said "I can only be your friend." He told me to apply what I had learned and by doing that I would stay within my Dharma (Life path). Even though I had spent years working on myself, his words jolted me and I felt suddenly disoriented. I felt disconnected and frightened. I hadn't been aware until then how dependent on him I had become. I saw at that moment that I still needed his support because I still felt fragmented. I still felt that important pieces of the puzzle were missing. After we separated, the nagging feeling of being incomplete pushed me onward and a short time later I joined the Pentecostal Church. Soon I began studying to become a minister, and when my studies were complete I went to the Dominican Republic to work as a missionary.

The I AM Within Me

The Pentecostal Church, unlike most modern Christian denominations, believes that even in the modern world the gifts of the spirit (healing, miracles, prophecy, etc.) are still being poured out through the Holy Spirit's indwelling, but that the Holy Spirit enters a person at a specific moment when a person consciously accepts Christ into their life. This is called a born-again experience. Although I could accept most of what I learned while I was in the Church, it was puzzling to me before and while I was a minister, how through a formula or ceremony in a church or even one experience or catharsis, a person could be converted from being spiritually dead, being disconnected from Christ (the universal field), to being spiritually alive, born again (reconnected to the universal field); in other words to remember who they were, recollect all the pieces and experience reunion. The process never made sense to me. It was too mechanical—one moment you're spiritually dead and the next moment you're spiritually alive.

I began to understand what was meant by rebirth and what true reunion meant only when I began using prayer as a tool for breaking energy blockages and making contact with the I AM within me. Prayer became a tool for my remembrance, recollection and reunion. As a mental and emotional release, and for the release of energy blockages, deep devotional prayer has no equal. Once I began to pray regularly, the barriers which kept me from experiencing the free radiation of mental and emotional energy began to crumble. As I poured out my deepest fears, pains, disappointments, I recovered lost parts of myself. As my heart softened, the second attention became more active. The more active it became, the more wholeness and unconditional joy I began to experience.

But my prayer life was not without crisis. In hindsight, I now see that the crises I experienced were always caused by my frustration at feeling incomplete, and it was my discomfort of feeling incomplete more than anything else which drove me onward. It drove me because deep within me was the desire to feel more whole, more connected to my body and more connected to the physical world. I was tired of being a sleepwalker, insensitive to the extraordinary world around me. As the blockages began to crumble, my prayers began to resonate from deep within me and the locked doors began to open. As the barriers came down, I began to experience another persona from deep within me, praying through me.

At first I wasn't sure what was going on, yet I knew it wasn't someone else praying through me because there was something familiar about the persona, about the frequencies of energy flowing through me when this persona expressed itself during times of prayer. I knew I had experienced the same fullness in childhood, the same feeling that I had grown rounder and larger. As I prayed in this way, I filled the environment with my presence and my relationship to everything seemed to change.

The feeling was one of deja-vu because on the edges of my conscious mind, I could remember experiences like it from early childhood. This persona, when I allowed it to express itself, grew in strength. As it expressed itself, waves of energy would rhythmically wash through my body filling me with inexpressible joy. This persona manifested itself in many ways; it took on different shapes, forms and personalities. Sometimes it expressed itself with gravity, sometimes with joy. In a short time, as I permitted this inner persona to express itself in its fullness, it became more integrated into my everyday life. Or perhaps it is more accurate to say I became more integrated into its life. It expressed itself through words during times of prayer, but also through the energy and expanded sense of self which began to pervade me.

The expanded vision and sense of self which resulted from this breakthrough changed my life. As this persona began to pervade my being, my fears began to dissipate and an inner strength began to pervade me, because my joy came from within and was no longer subject to the vagaries of my outer experiences. At last, I had come home. At last I remembered who I was, and through recollection and re-union I finally experienced myself as an integrated human being; the synthesis of selves; the "I AM."

Tagore, the Indian poet, echoed this when he wrote in *Gitanjali*:

> The traveller has to know at every alien door to come to his own, and one has to wander through all the outer worlds to reach the innermost shrine at the end. My eyes strayed far and wide before I shut them and said into tears of thousand streams and deluge the world with the flood of the assurance "I AM."[1]

Going Within

The emergence of the I AM, which is the result of psychospiritual integration, is a natural process that goes on undisturbed in a person whose energy system is free of blockages and barriers. It is natural and requires no effort to sustain because it is supported by the "ALL," higher consciousness, who eternally seeks union with his/her creation. While I was in the church, Jesus served as an archetype for me much as the Bodhisattva or avatar does in the East. He was for me the living proof that each of us can remember and recollect ourselves; reunite the separate parts of our being and become whole again.

But it must be understood by any sincere student that wholeness can only be achieved by seeing into the nature of one's being, accepting it as it is and permitting it the liberty to express itself naturally. As each person permits themselves this liberty, they deliver themselves from slavery into freedom. If a person hopes to achieve wholeness by looking outside themselves for some Messiah or magical formula, their search becomes vain and their goal impossible to achieve. Only by looking within can a person again experience the liberation of all the natural energy and power which has been imprisoned within them, which under their fragmented way of living has become squashed and distorted, and instead of being expressed naturally as it should be, it can only be expressed abnormally. When a person begins looking within, they soon find evidence of their true nature and inherent complexity. As they probe into the root of their being, their nature reveals itself in its fullness. They begin to see that they are far more than they had hitherto imagined. They begin to see that in every direction they border the infinite.

The Whole Self

In the metaphor below, a young Brahman (the arche-

busco

typical student) for years sought peace ... he sought release from the constant suffering he experienced. Unlike other youths of his age who knew what they wanted, he sought only one thing: release from his constant torment. On his path he met many people who sympathized with his suffering and who offered him either advice or comfort. But neither helped him for any length of time. At the point of despair he learned of a wise man who had become whole, who had achieved peace.

He was told that the wise man lived deep in the forest. After an arduous journey, he found the sage sitting by a small stream under an old banyan tree. The old man invited him to sit down. After a while the seeker found the courage to ask: "How shall I become whole and thereby achieve peace?"

The teacher gazed at him and after a few moments spoke. "Go to the village and there you will find what you seek."

The young man thanked the sage and then quickly left for the village, full of hope and expectation. But when he arrived at the village he found only some huts and three old women sitting in the marketplace with baskets in front of them. One was selling pieces of wood, another pieces of metal and the last, wire. With his last coins the Brahman bought a piece of metal, a piece of wood, a piece of metal and a length of wire thinking that perhaps they had some magical properties. But he soon saw that there was nothing magical about them. They were quite ordinary. Disappointed, he returned to the sage and told him what he found. He scolded the sage and demanded an explanation for being deceived.

All the sage would say was, "You will soon understand."

Dejected, the young Brahman departed and with nowhere to go he wandered through the forest. After a time when his anger and disappointment began to fade, he heard the sound of music coming through the wood. Since it was growing dark, he hurried in the direction of the music. As he drew closer he could hear that it came from a sitar. Deeply moved, he allowed himself to be drawn to the music.

To his surprise he discovered that the music was being played by the sage who earlier had made a fool of him. Moreover, to his amazement, he realized that in his wanderings he had gone in circles and had returned to the very spot where he left the old man. It was then that he became aware of the sage's fingers which played with amazing dexterity. He became so transfixed that for a moment he forgot himself, and in that very instant a flash of insight burst upon him. He saw that the sitar was made out of wood, metal and wire.

In that instant, the old man's message became clear to him. He realized for the first time that as long as he considered the wood, metal and wire separately they held no significance for him. But when he put them together and saw them as a whole, they became a sitar. He now saw the wisdom of the sage's teaching. He had been given everything he needed.

From the moment he was born, he was complete; whole in every way. He had not realized that the different facets of his being were never meant to be picked apart. Instead they were part of a complex ecology of spirit, soul and body which together formed a whole being. For the first time he grasped that each separate piece could be understood only when viewed as part of the whole. In the past he had been obsessed with the separate pieces of himself and identifying with one and rejecting the others he had become lost. Until this moment of recognition he had never realized that to identify with any one aspect of his being was to lose the significance of the others and to lose sight of who he really was. He saw at last that life is a process of remembrance, recollection and finally reunion.

Herman Hesse grasped the importance of integration when he wrote: Siddhartha (near the end of his life) listened attentively to the river and heard the . . . "song of a thousand voices; when he did not listen to the sorrow or laughter, when he did not bind his soul to any one particular voice and absorb it in his self, but heard them all, the whole, the unity; then the great song of a thousand voices consisted of one word: Om-perfection."[2]

CHAPTER VI

FEAR AND PRANA

... be steady in truth, free from worldly anx-
ieties and centered in the self.
—*Bhagavad Gita*

Wholeness, which is the goal of psychospiritual integration, cannot be achieved when fear stands in the way and
blocks it. Fear is self-limiting, fear makes a person feel fee-
ble, small and ultimately insecure. It causes a person to contract on every level, it disrupts the energy system and the
relationship he/she has to themselves and to everyone else.

There are many sorts of fear, and volumes have been
written about it. Ultimately, fear is the antithesis of being,
and at the root of all fear is the fear of non-being. The
ultimate fear is not the fear of death but rather extinction,
total lovelessness which is the ultimate separation.

When we experience ourselves as whole, as part of the
great ecology that is the synthesis of everything in the visible and invisible universe, the universal field, we soon see
that extinction is impossible. The Hermetic philosophy*

---

* Hermetics originated in ancient Egypt. We are told that it was given to mankind by Thoth
the Egyptian god of wisdom who the Greeks later called Hermes Trismegistus. He was hailed
from the earliest times as the "Master of Masters." If Hermes did exist, he is truly the father of
esoteric wisdom. The details of his life have been lost to us, but one tradition has it that he was
a contemporary of Abraham's. Whatever the truth may be, Hermes gave man a set of
teachings which have influenced philosophy and religion ever since.

tells us "the universe as a whole, and in its parts or unity, has its existence in the Mind of the ALL, in which mind we live, move and have our being."[1] The unconditional radiation of energy we call the ALL connects everything. It is the great unifying force which radiates throughout all planes of causation. It is the force that pulls together, that builds bridges, that builds relationship, that binds the universe together . . . it is the unifying principle which binds matter, energy and consciousness on all planes.

As energy-concentrates, we are integral parts of the universal field of energy and we can no more be removed from it than a stitch can be removed from knitting without the knitting being unraveled. As long as we consciously allow ourselves to radiate freely, we will consciously experience the joy of being connected to the rest of the universal field. By blocking the free radiation of energy because of contraction which results from fear, we lose the conscious sense of security and contentment which only can come from that experience. It is then that we feel truly separate and alone.

Da Free John writes:

Fear opposed to love (the universal consciousness) which is free feeling—radiation—is the tendency towards contraction of one's whole being. It is the tendency to become separate, to pull oneself out of the universal field of energy and consciousness. Fear fills the vacuum created by the absence of relationship, caused by . . . separation. Whenever the individual is in relationship to life . . . then fear cannot arise.[2]

As long as fear keeps a person fragmented and separate from everyone else, and as long as a person believes in the gospel of separation, not believing and experiencing union and true intimacy, which grows out of love, as long as they still strive against everyone else and ignore the promoting of the I AM, which forever seeks union, they will remain an island, locked into the vicious circle of competition striving against "others" outside themselves and the "others" buried within their unconscious. They will ultimately mistrust everyone, as well as themselves, and will live in silent fear ultimately insecure and alone.

Not Being

When we talk of the fear of extinction, we must ask ourselves who within us is afraid of extinction. Is it the I AM which fears separation and extinction, or is it some other part of self which fears it and throws up a wall of fear when its existence is threatened? Where there is certainty, there is no fear. Fear comes when there is doubt, where the outcome is unsure. There can be no fear where the I AM is concerned, because there is no doubt experienced by the I AM as to its continuated existence and its relationship to the universal energy field which permeates the universe.

In the final analysis, the I AM is without fear, because in a world of endless transmutation, it knows that life and death are simply transitions from one level of causation to another, one reality to another. The I AM extinction is inconceivable because it knows that nothing that exists within the universal field can cease to be; its outer form may change, it may move up or down on the evolutionary scale by having its vibrations altered, but the primal fear of extinction, the existential despair of complete separation, is impossible.

Lord Shri Krishna tells prince Arjuna in the Bhagavad Gita "the wise grieve neither for the dead nor for the living. There was never a time when I was not, nor thou, nor these princes were not; there will never be a time when we shall cease to be."[3]

Moreover, in the Upanishads we read:

in the beginning there existed only self . . .
He examined everywhere and could not see
anything but himself.
He was scared
That is why even today one gets scared
When one stays alone
The Great Being contemplated,
When there is nothing else
but me. Then whom shall I be afraid of?
When he thus thought, his fear was removed
Because really whom could he fear?
He had no second; it is only when there
Is a second, that one is afraid

The I AM, the union of selves, is forever in union with the universal field. The I AM's relationship to the universal field can be likened to a wave which is part of the sea (the universal energy field) owes its existence to the sea, but manifests its individuality by rising from the pool and asserting power, form and even generating energy before it returns to the sea after its term is complete. Its understanding is intuitive. It learns by immersing itself in what it experiences. It touches what it experiences and allows itself to be touched in return. In this way it experiences directly and fully.

Moreover, the certainty of survival eludes consciousness (the rational mind and the physical body and its senses) because it has no roots. Its existence is always threatened because it is not immersed in the universal field of energy. It lies on the surface of the universal field rather than floating in it. It is supported by the field like a boat floating on the sea, but it is nonetheless not part of the field.

Since it is not immersed in the universal field, the consciousness, in order to understand something, must examine it with the first attention from some point of reference. It can only understand other structures in terms of itself, in terms of past experience. It must break the universe up and analyze it in order to understand it. By its very nature, consciousness sees the trees but not the forest. By relying on the senses and rational mind, consciousness can only understand the universe one part at a time. Consciousness can be thought of as the visible part of a person. It is intellectual, rational, and its active orientation is toward the physical world. It is "action" intensive, which means that it fills its time and space with doing; which can be anything from thinking and feeling to building or destroying.

Ego shares in both: consciousness and unconsciousness. Ego in its purest form is the synthesis interrelating centers of awareness and energy.

The Ego

A person's point of contact with the world is the ego. The ego derives its form from the conscious nature which is "me" centered and which experiences everything outside itself as the "other" and from I AM which is the unconscious nature, and experiences everything as part of the universal whole where everything is united and there is no "other."

When the ego rests at the middle point so that it participates in the unconscious nature as well as the conscious nature it is aware that its existence is within the "All," and like the I AM it is aware that this relationship can never be broken.

However, when the ego develops exclusively within consciousness, this certainly eludes it because by developing within consciousness alone it has no roots securing it to the universal field.

When ego rests exclusively in consciousness, it does not perform its natural function which is to be a bridge between consciousness and unconsciousness, the rational and intuitive . . . . the visible world and the invisible world.

The diagram below illustrates this.

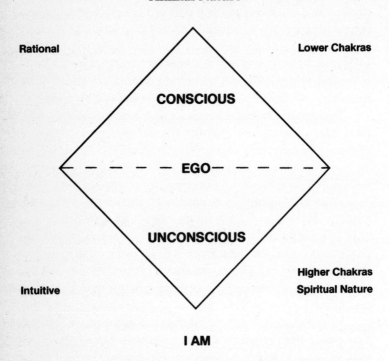

Animal Nature

Rational   Lower Chakras

CONSCIOUS

← — — — EGO — — — — →

UNCONSCIOUS

                                            Higher Chakras
Intuitive   Spiritual Nature

I AM

If the ego is trapped in consciousness, then free radiation of the I AM through unconsciousness becomes restricted. In this condition a person will identify with consciousness alone because their ego, their point of contact to the manifest world is trapped within it. This automatically makes a person fearful because they lose awareness of the I AM, the eternal part of themselves. A person in this condition becomes motivated by "me" concerns because there are no deep roots extending into unconsciousness. Everything has a superficiality about it.

Without deep roots extending into unconsciousness, a person becomes alienated from the unconscious selves. When this happens, a person appears to be dominated by the ego, but it would be more accurate to say that their ego is dominated by consciousness. Consciousness sees the rest of the universe including the I AM as outside itself—as something to be feared—as separate energy and separate centers of awareness. Because of its fear of extinction, it sees its separate identity as something to be defended, and it will use its power to exclude the I AM from participation in ego and will try to usurp the ego for itself.

Detachment

Fear is used by consciousness to maintain its pre-eminent position. Wherever it is threatened, whenever the I AM asserts itself through ego, consciousness throws up a wall of fear. The more identified a person is with their conscious life, the more effective the device becomes. It has become so effective in most people's life that the mere threat of its use is sufficient to keep the I AM imprisoned and keep it under the heavy yoke of consciousness. But the fear brandished by consciousness is based on attachment and desire, and that is its chief weakness. The more attached a person is to their conscious life, and this can be translated into the more they need and desire, the more their behavior will be controlled by fear.

Once a person breaks the habit of attachment and begins the process of psychospiritual integration by allowing the unconscious parts to emerge, they break the vicious hold that this fear has over them. They can then root themselves in the I AM and break out of the circle of desire and fear. This new posture becomes possible because they experience a greater reality, a greater security, and as a result their fears and desires quickly lose their influence over them.

A person who has achieved detachment cannot be

coerced by fear into accepting the authority of consciousness, because the individual has inner resources which
nourish him. The consciousness has nothing of value to
offer someone whose needs are already met in other ways,
who has seen that at the root of his being he is complete,
whole, who continually experiences unconditional love
flowing into him from the universal field.

Fearlessness

A whole person is not controlled by fear. He betrays
fearlessness at every turn, not in words, but in his whole
demeanor: one has only to look at him to see it. To be free
from fear does not mean pretending to yourself that you are
fearless or consciously courageous. Rather he who masters
his fear of extinction is free from fear of any kind to the
extent that he is no longer capable of experiencing what
fear feels like. This passage from *Hagakure*, which dates
from about the middle of the 17th century explains:

> Yagyu Tajima-no-kami was a great swordsman
> and teacher in the court of Shogun of the time, Tokugawa
> Iyamitsu. One of the personal guards of the Shogun
> one day came to Tajima-no-kami wishing to be trained
> in fencing. The master said "As I observe you seem to
> be a master of fencing yourself, pray tell me what
> school you belong, before we enter relationship of
> teacher and pupil."
>
> The guardsman said, "I am ashamed to confess
> that I have never learned the art."
>
> "Are you going to fool me? I am teacher to the
> honorable Shogun himself and I know my judging
> eye never fails."
>
> "I am sorry to defy your honour, but I really know
> nothing." This resolute denial on the part of the visitor
> made the swordmaster think for awhile and he finally
> said: "If you say so, it must be so; but still I am sure you
> are a master of something, though I do not know of
> what."
>
> "If you insist, I will tell you. There is one thing of

which I can say I am complete master. When I was still a boy, the thought came upon me that as a Samurai I ought in no circumstances to be afraid of death, and I have grappled with the problem of death now for some years, and finally the problem of death ceased to worry me. May this be at what you hint?"

"Exactly," exclaimed Tajima-no-kami. "That is what I mean. I am glad that I made no mistake in my judgment. For the ultimate secrets of swordsmanship also lie in being released from the thought of death. I have trained ever so many hundreds of my pupils along this line, but so far none of them really deserve the final certificate for swordsmanship. You need no technical training, you are already a master."

The Samurai's mastery of fear was the essential element in his mastery of swordsmanship. In the same way, finding the courage and honesty to face one's fears is an essential step on the path to becoming whole again.

Angela's story is an example of what can happen when one has the courage to face their fears directly.

"There—that's it, you've got it, stay in that space. You're experiencing wholeness." I was sitting there talking with Keith about some of my attitudes and games that keep me from really feeling alive and joyful. My first reaction to his exclamation was, "Is that what he calls wholeness? Everybody knows this state, this feeling, it can't be that simple."

I felt very strong at that moment, strong and soft at the same time, it really felt like me—but a me I hadn't experienced in a long time. It began with a feeling of personal strength and self-confidence but it grew into a state that involved much more than that.

I could feel a glowing sensation inside myself. It was a feeling of being lifted up and at the same time having been rooted profoundly, it was really the feeling of expanding and filling space with myself. This glowing sensation was so strong that I just had to pour it out. It was a moment of absolute inner peacefulness, but full of sparkling energy at the same time. A new dimension of my being opened to me. Only months ago I wasn't even aware that one could actually feel this way as an adult. Before I met Keith I could hardly even feel my physical body let alone the inner joy which radiated from some deep place within me. My body had always been just a substance which moved as a whole, but inner sensations I had never felt. I had never paid any attention to sensations inside the body, it has been completely numb and dark and that state was all I knew.

By doing the exercises Keith recommended regularly, and starting to pay attention to changes inside my body, I started to get a glimpse of how sensitive our bodies can be. But actually not until that night did I or better my body fully wake up to that reality. Something was breathing, pulsating, vibrating, tingling, sparkling inside me and it was joyful and exciting. I no longer felt contracted, fearful. My doubt was transformed into joy. For the first time in years I was able to reach out into the environment. The degree to which people affect each other only then became clear to me. During the time I was being truly myself, I became consciously aware of the messages that we get from other people. We communicate with each other all the time, but we are normally not aware of it. Now that I could feel myself I could consciously project energy and messages to others, consciously reach out and communicate with another person on a nonverbal level. It is unbelievably beautiful and exciting to communicate in this way.

Another truly amazing thing is what happens to your mind. Usually my mind is always in action, thinking, worrying, wondering, fearing, etc. From the moment I began experiencing with my whole self, my mind became absolutely clear. For the first time I realized that I really didn't need those thoughts floating through my mind.

The moment I fell into the state of wholeness all the qualities of that state became clear to me. Before that, I had understood rationally what wholeness was about—living without fear, being yourself at every moment—but I had the misleading notion that once you obtain it, you have it and cannot lose it, like a secure harbor where all fear and anxiety would cease to exist. I could look at it from all sides and grasp it rationally, but inside I didn't feel it, I didn't sense it. Now I had become it. Everything looked the same, but everything had changed. It was as if a veil had been lifted from my face: I saw that we must choose to radiate and be ourselves completely, every moment of the day.

We all know this space, but we choose to let it go. It is more comfortable and undemanding to live the way we always lived. For me, I had chosen to be a "good girl" rather than myself. The extent to which that pattern was rooted in me and shaped my life only became clear to me when I experienced my wholeness. Deep down in me there was a feeling of not being lovable, of not being worth anything the way I was, I always felt I had to do something in order to be worth something. Love was not unconditional, joyful, giving, but conditional, demanding, possessive. Being was not enough, doing became the key to my getting love and feeling love.

In daily life it meant for me that my self-esteem and contentment did not come from within, but I had to seek it from outside, namely in relationships with other people. I had to overcome the fear of being judged and rejected. But once I did overcome my fear, life became unimaginably exciting, magical and joyful.

CHAPTER VII

BLOOMING AGAIN

Children do not give up their innate imagination, curiosity, dreaminess easily, you have to
love them to get them to do that.

—R. D. Laing

Tagore, the great Indian mystic and poet wrote: "He whom
I enclose with my name is weeping in this dungeon. I am
ever busy building this wall all around; and as this wall goes
up into the sky day by day, I lost sight of my true being in its
dark shadow. I take pride in this great wall, and I plaster it
with dust and sand, lest a least hole should be left in this
name: and for all the care I take I lose sight of my true
being."[1]

Because of blockages and fragmentation caused by
fear, the vast majority of people have lost the experience of
unconditional joy and union with the universal field. A person's experience of unconditional joy depends on their
access to unconsciousness and the multitude of selves contained within it.

Plato in the *Phaedrus* says that the soul of man is imprisoned in his physical body (and consciousness) . . . like
an oyster in its shell, and Elizabeth Haisch tells us that
"From the time a self dwells in it, the body develops a

power of resistance corresponding to the average degree of consciousness of the spirit dwelling in it."[2]

Loss of unconditional joy and union with the universal field begins in early childhood. Studies suggest that pain and fear, which can lead to fragmentation and the loss of unconditional joy, can even begin during gestation. Dr. Arthur Janov writes, "What is happening throughout pre- and postuterine life is that there are stresses which are leaving their marks on the organism, forming a primal pool which one day overflows into symptoms"[3], i.e. fragmentation. The fetus (on an unconscious level) is aware of changes in its environment, both its physical environment, which is the mother's womb and physical body, as well as the psychic environment which includes to a large extent the inner environment of the mother; her energy level, emotional maturity, her level of stress and her mental and emotional condition.

Symbiosis

Since the fetus and later the infant is so dependent on the physical and psychic condition of the mother, we can say that prior to birth and for several months after birth there is a symbiosis physically and energetically between mother and child. Union exists or should exist between the two. However, this union can be disrupted. And this in effect will disrupt the child's personal energy field and its relationship to the universal field. Something as seemingly innocent as a mother's attitude can affect the energy bond between the child and mother. Sensations in the mother affect her unborn child energetically while it is still in the womb.

Janov postulates that sensations experienced by the fetus, especially in the later stages of development, are the precursers of feelings. Moreover, catastrophic sensations experienced by the mother can disrupt the relationship between mother and fetus on the interpersonal as well as energy level. The child's energy system before and a short time after birth is fully integrated with the mother's, and in essence the child's experiences of the world are filtered through the mother's energy system.

Pregnancy

If during pregnancy, labor, and delivery the newborn is subject to stresses which are the result of both psychic shock as well as physical shock, these can develop into full grown neurosis later.

Imbalances in a mother's hormone system while she is pregnant can cause changes in the fetus which can have a lifelong effect. Such changes in the fetus can determine how passive or assertive a child will be. It can affect his will, the quality of his relationships and shape his self-image. These physical problems reflect imbalances in the child's subtle energy system which suggests that even before birth a child can develop energy blockages, imbalances in Yin (feminine) and Yang (masculine) energy, or suffer a disruption in the subtle energy system's ability to distribute, store and sense energy. It may even affect how right brained or left brained the child is, which means how intuitive or rational the child will become.

Research has linked imbalance in the mother's hormone system (which can be caused by fear, anxiety or emotional strain due to repressed feelings) to how aggressive or passive a child will become. A study in which male hormones were administered to pregnant primates resulted in more aggressive offspring than the control group.

The aggressive behavior remained consistent and persisted throughout adulthood. In another study, male rats were administered the female hormone estrogen just after being born. They acquired female behavior which persisted during their whole life. Another group that was given estrogen later (several weeks after birth) did not experience the same persistent feminization.

Childbirth

The moment of childbirth is a crucial one for the child. The experiences at the moment of birth profoundly affect the energy system, relationships and one's later development.

The moment the child chooses to enter the world is not a matter of chance, it is a function of the fetus' relationship to its mother's energy field as well as the universal field. The precise time of birth therefore is a function of the interaction of energy fields in various rhythms. Some of these rhythms are biological and some are subtle rhythms determined by the ebb and flow of subtle energy.

Research has shown us that on every level of life from bacteria to mullocks, from cats and dogs to baboons and men, rhythms of work and repose forced on us by the hours of light and darkness correspond to the rhythms inherent in the cells themselves. This was recognized long ago by the prophets and sages. The fifth Hermetic axiom states: "everything flows, out and in: everything has its tides; all things rise and fall, the pendulum swing manifests in everything; the measure of the swing to the right is the measure of the swing to the left; rhythm compensates."[4]

In more modern times, the biologist Gay Luce tells us: "it is abundantly clear that healthy living things are not only internally rhythmic; they are also synchronized with their environment."[5]

The process of childbirth is no less subject to the universal laws of rhythm. However, since the Industrial Revolution, women in Western society have increasingly moved away from the natural rhythmic childbirth of the lower animals. They have forgotten the natural rhythms as their lives have become more disjointed and separated from the natural flow which for ages they had instinctively obeyed.

In modern times, women are taught how to give birth with the result that their natural rhythm is disrupted, and this disrupts the relationship and energy flow between mother and child at the crucial moment the child chooses to enter the world.

Moreover, most women who come to the hospital to give birth are soon drugged so that they become a non-person and as such don't participate in the birth of the child. They are brought down to the level of a machine; they can't respond naturally and their natural rhythms are disrupted. Even worse, because of the drugs they are given, they cannot feel their body or their baby's body, and as a result their child is cut off from the energy support of the mother which she would give consciously and unconsciously if she were not drugged. Before the baby is even out of the birth canal, its natural rhythms and its relationship to its mother's energy field and to the universal field has been disrupted. At the moment of birth, the child is plucked from the warmth and security of its mother and her energy field and its first experience of the physical world is the pain of separation. Janov tells us the mother's condition during birth (if she is drugged or contracted) . . . "is a literal adversity for the fetus. Just to come alive he must overcome it. He is in a struggle before he breathes his first breath. No matter how many facts are in her head, no matter how well she is trained for childbirth . . . If a mother has shut down, and if those repressions are mediated by tense musculature, then when pain strikes again in childbirth, the musculature (of which the uterus and vaginal canal are part) will automatically respond by clamping down."[6]

Janov calls this syndrome the birth trauma. The birth trauma can be particularly devastating to the child energetically. During delivery, the child is being removed from the physical and energetic embrace of its mother for the first time. Those births in which the child is physically taken away from the mother right after birth are most disruptive, because the child is alone outside the aura of the mother. When removed more than 20 centimeters from the mother, the child is outside the protective umbrella of the mother's etheric aura*. When the child is within the mother's etheric aura, there is an unconscious rhythmic flow of love and emotional energy from mother to child. If the child is taken outside the mother's etheric aura, it loses contact with the mother emotionally. When the child is removed more than two and a half meters from the mother, the child loses contact on the mental level as well because the child is outside the mother's mental aura or mental field. In these cases, there is no contact on the unconscious, mental level, and unless the mother thinks directly about her child, there will be no contact on the conscious, mental level either. When outside the emotional mental fields of the mother, it is the mother who must consciously reach out for the child emotionally and mentally in order to keep contact. The child cannot reach out for the mother simply because it has not yet developed the facilities to do so. If the mother is drugged she will be unable to retain contact with her child, and if she is ego-centered or afraid and doesn't consciously reach out for the child after it is taken from her, this will compound the child's first experience of separation, aloneness and pain. If the pain is too severe, it will overload the child's energy system and the child will not be able to process and release the catastrophic feelings it is experiencing.

Infancy

If the infant's connection to its parents is disrupted after birth because of energy blockages in one of the parents, the infant's personal energy field will continue to be disrupted.

---

* Each person has three auras which surround the body: the etheric aura, mental aura and spiritual aura. They are reservoirs of subtle energy which are part of a person's personal energy field.

This will have a negative effect on the child's ego development whose roots should reach deep down into unconsciousness. If the ego develops primarily within consciousness, the child will never attain full emotional maturity and this will prevent them from having mature relationships later. It can even preclude the basic understanding of what a natural mature human relationship is like.

The following story of F. gives insight into the difficulties one must overcome when proper ego development has been disrupted.

My mother was an unwed mother and my father was an alcoholic. My mother gave birth to me in a home for single mothers.

When I reached the age of two, my mother got married after having given birth to her third child. I experienced some family life with my mother, my stepfather and my sister. However, this lasted only for a short while. Then my sister was taken to an aunt and I was taken to my grandparents. Later I was given to foster parents. As a child I was totally confused as to where I belonged and who to trust. I was wild and difficult, my foster parents kept me for one year, then they decided that they didn't want to keep me any longer. As a child I suffered from a speech defect as well as nightmares.

After the third year of school, the teachers and my parents decided that I was too slow to follow ordinary classes and I should go to a children's home where I lived and went to school for about one year. I kept being pushed backwards and forwards up to the age of 15 when I lived again with my mother and stepfather. My fits of anger and aggression in childhood slowly turned into depression with puberty. By age 15 I was taking drugs. During the following two years, I felt very unstable and often changed my place of living. Most of the time I was loaded with drugs, and one day I attempted suicide which resulted in injuries to my back. After this, I was put into an institution for recalcitrant girls where they tried to guide me back into a normal life. Later, a therapeutic community was set up in my town and I was brought there. I was full of mistrust, wild and shrewish at first. I was told that I only had two alternatives: either to stay in this community and behave or I would be brought to juvenile prison. I decided to stay in the community. After a little while, I began to experience a real change in my life because I was forced to live together with other people and to talk to them in group therapy. I lived for three years in this community and during that time, I realized that life was worth living. Later I met a man with whom I fell in love but my feelings of jealousy, envy and the fear of being rejected as well as the need to possess someone were so strong and I finally destroyed the relationship.

In 1985, somebody told me about an American healer who was teaching in Europe. After a certain hesitation, I decided to become one of his students in order to learn more about his work with chakras and energy. But even though I began working with him, I continued to move according to my old patterns. It took me a long time to realize that there are no structures and patterns with a spiritual teacher. Everything is open—every day is another day. But I was attached to having a situation, a surrounding that gave me security and since he wouldn't give this to me I started to project my misery outside and made others responsible for my discomfort, my fears and my despair.

More and more I felt like I was torn in two parts. I was longing to discover a state of absolute devotion, love and detachment but noticed at the same time that I could not open up because I feared to be rejected. I could not admit that I loved somebody because I did not trust my feelings. After weeks of confusion I went to Keith and he told me that the only way out of my personal crisis was to break the blockages which kept me from loving myself unconditionally. He told me I must examine my attitude toward him, toward energy work and toward myself. I suffered for hours asking myself repeatedly the question: what does he mean? I tried to figure out what my motives and attitudes were and where they came from. I finally reached a point where there was only one possibility: drop the past and live in the present.

So I started to meditate regularly and to pay attention to the way I carried my body, to where I felt tensions and to whether my energy was flowing properly. Within a short time I felt changes in my whole energy system. I felt my heart open and it became easier to react appropriately toward people. I rediscovered what I have been longing for the whole time, love—the love that Keith had explained to me was possible when I became whole again by being completely myself.

Sucking

An infant's connection and relationship to its mother is predicated on its needs to attain physical and psychic nourishment from her. If the child can't energetically give and take freely from its mother, if the baby can't project its needs to her, its energy system will be disrupted. In the case of nursing, a baby is born with a need to suck and with the instinctive ability to do so. If a child is inadequately breast-fed or not breast-fed at all, the child can be wounded psychologically and energetically by not getting the time needed for sucking. This can disrupt the energy moving through the child's shoulders, neck and mouth. (The region of the shoulders, neck and mouth are regulated by the fifth chakra.) The pain of not securing sufficient time or comfort during sucking will cause a contraction in the baby's fifth chakra. This contraction will be transmuted into the physical body which will result in the contraction of the shoulder, neck, throat and mouth muscles. The physical contraction will cause a further restriction of energy. Contraction of the fifth chakra has a serious effect on the child because the fifth chakra controls self-expression, which means the expression of thoughts and emotions verbally and non-verbally, as well as the total expression of the physical body. The baby's ability to move spontaneously, joyfully, and rhythmically is also regulated by the fifth chakra. Moreover, the fifth chakra is a watershed where all feelings coming up from the lower body are transmuted into joy. When the chakra is traumatized and blocked in infancy, the child will grow up with an inability to process (to transmute into joy and release) the strong feelings of pain, fear and anger. As a result, these feelings get stuck in the subtle energy system and they form the reservoirs of pain, fear and anger which get walled off and lead to fragmentation. The more difficulty the infant has in processing feelings, the more easily the child will be overloaded and the more introverted the child will become. In the most extreme cases the child will either choose a fantasy world where every pain, fearful situation or angry word becomes magnified beyond the child's ability to process it, or the child will choose to disintegrate completely into multiple personalities. In multiple personalities, the "selves" work completely independently. Brainwave patterns, handedness, and allergies differ as multiple personalities shift. Therapists report scores of bizarre symptoms experienced by multiples. One therapist reported that a female patient had three menstrual periods each month—one for each of her personalities. Another multiple required different prescription eye glasses for his different ego "states."[7]

Frank Puntram, psychiatrist and psychologist at the Natural Institute of Mental Health, said: "Multiples seem to vary as much from one personality to another as from one normal person to another."[8]

Toilet Training, Etc.

When a child's free radiation of energy is disrupted during the period of toilet training, there is often a disruption of energy flowing through the first chakra at the base of the spine. The first chakra roots a person to the Earth and makes him feel fundamentally secure. When the energy of the first chakra is blocked, frequencies of energy associated with survival, security and safety will be blocked. If the child doesn't feel these feelings internally, he will spend his life seeking them outside himself, often through acquiring food, possessions, etc. which makes him feel safe.

If there is a lack of sensory stimulation by the parents, if the parents have difficulty feeling their own body and expressing affection, if the child isn't sufficiently cuddled or it it is allowed to cry itself to sleep, there will be a disruption in the second chakra. Disruption in the second chakra will make it difficult for the child to feel his own physical body and in a short while he will become physically insensitive and numb. In this situation, the child is conditioned to develop a passive personality. The numbness often forces the child into a life dominated by sensual pleasures. There is the tendency to see people as objects useful for gratifying desires only. When there is disruption in either the first or second chakra, a person becomes dependent on the outside world for his happiness and he tries everything to satisfy the lack of sensation within his own body and subtle energy system. When something that gives pleasure is withdrawn, there is often a deep feeling of emptiness which is caused by the lack of sensation in the body and lack of energy, since sexual energy and Kundalini* are both restricted. This kind of disruption can begin any time from birth to puberty. At puberty the disruption is often more acute since the flow of sexual energy is stronger during the period of sexual maturation. Disruption at puberty can lead to all forms of sexual dysfunction since blockages involving the first and second chakra prevent sexual energy from flowing properly past the second chakra and through the appropriate channels.

---

* Kundalini—the serpent energy, located at the base of the spine. It is considered to be the most powerful stream of subtle energy in a human being.

Conditional Love

As the child grows older, he becomes more independent. He becomes less dependent on the mother and her energy system. The child begins to explore its world and comes into contact first with other members of the family, then with people outside the family unit. Difficulties within the immediate family can disrupt the child's energy system and the child's ability to remain whole or engage in intimate relationships within the family or later with friends, colleagues, spouse and children. When love is given by the parents conditionally or contractually, i.e. I will love you if you are good, if you are pretty, if you love me back, then there is an implicit message given with the love. That message is "You are not good enough as you are." There is nothing more catastrophic for a child than the loss of parental love. The younger the child is, the more catastrophic the loss is. When forced to make the choice between the loss of parental love or the rejection of a part of "self," the child will usually agree with the parent and reject part of themselves as not good enough rather than lose the parent's love.

Rejecting an essential part of self has a profound effect on the child energetically. It will inhibit the free radiation of energy coming through consciousness and unconsciousness and will help create "little demons," the "others," which first the parent rejected, then the child rejects. The problem is that these demons became demons only because they were rejected and received no love. The more they are rejected, the darker they become and the more they will torment the child and later the adult, until they are finally let out of their prison (within the unconscious), accepted and given the love they needed.

Anger

Anger within the family, even if not directed toward the child, will disrupt the child's energy system. Anger, like love, is an outward-going radiation. However, it is rarely expressed appropriately. It usually is tinged with judgments such as you are bad, or there is something wrong with you. If the anger radiated freely, it would simply be a momentary burst of energy and would express only the angry person's discomfort. It would sound something like "Stop doing that" or, "I don't like what you are doing." Since it is rarely expressed in this way, it causes both the angry person, the target and anyone else caught in the distorted energy field to contract. By expressing their anger inappropriately, parents inadvertently damage their child's energy system by subjecting him to a distorted energy field and by doing this, they disrupt their child's connection to the universal field. If the parents resent each other, if they are often angry and hostile, the child will be caught in the middle of this distorted energy field and when the child repeatedly finds himself in this situation, he will learn to restrict the free flow of his energy because by flowing outward, he encounters barriers which cause him pain. This scenario will ultimately break down the child's ability to trust.

Trust

Trust is the unconscious awareness that it is safe to radiate freely. The ability to trust allows a person the freedom to radiate without old fears getting in the way. It allows a person to feel ultimately secure. A breakdown of trust will alienate a person or make him dependent as he tries to find a safe place in a world he finds hostile and dangerous. Many people are not aware of their inability to trust.

A child's trust can be shattered when one or both parents use their child in a struggle for power against the other parent. A power struggle within the family is an ominous sign . . . indicating the breakdown of trust and love between husband and wife. "Where love reigns, there is no will to power; and where the will to power is paramount, love is lacking. The one is but the shadow of the other . . . "9

Normally, the child views the parents as protectors, but when one of the parents becomes the child's antagonist, there will be a disruption in the energy flowing between parent and child. This will disrupt the child's free radiation of energy. Often the child will fight fire with fire by asserting its own power, choosing power over love because of the antagonistic situation created by one of the parents. In the long run, the child invariably suffers. Moreover, they often find themself as an adult setting up the same "power games" that they learned as a child at home. Nothing will change this situation until a person breaks these blockages which restrict their normal energy flow so that it can again radiate freely.

If, as the child grows older, his ego develops without roots in the unconscious, the will to have power will grow stronger and the joyful feelings of energy flowing through the subtle energy system and the physical body will grow duller. The child will become an insensitive adult and the will to have power will make him even less powerful as the auric fields surrounding him become weakened because of the inability of his subtle energy system to transmute and distribute a healthy amount of energy. When this is the case, the child finds himself cut off from the I AM and he becomes hostile toward life . . . in particular his own inner life.

An ego that is out of touch with the unconscious is a dangerous thing. It turns against the I AM, the union of selves, and tries to inhibit it by creating an exaggerated sense of its self. It tries to create a single dominant persona "me," and it tries to identify exclusively with it. The ego rooted only in consciousness usurps the role of the I AM, locks a person into a linear universe which is superficial and is without depth and real love.

Innocence

A child's life is normally a magical time, because by not being fully developed consciousness has not yet usurped the position of the I AM and its vehicles, intuition and unconscious awareness.

In Yoga, the first seven years of a child's life are called the years of joy and innocence. Normally, energy flows unobstructed between the first and seventh chakra. There is little or no fragmentation, and as a result, a child enjoys the experience of union with the All. He lives a life of innocence entered in the now with no real understanding of past or future.

All children for varying lengths of time rest in the unconscious union with the universal field and enjoy the fruits which flow from it. Jesus acknowledged a child's privileged state when He said: "Suffer the little children to come unto me, and forbid them not: for of such is the Kingdom of God."[10] But as a child develops a separate identity as the concepts of I, you, mine, yours come into awareness, consciousness develops, and to the extent that ego is rooted in consciousness rather than unconsciousness, that is the extent that the child loses the sense of union with the All. The price of becoming conscious without maintaining a balance between unconscious and consciousness is the loss of conscious union with the All.

Using the biblical metaphor, we can say as long as a child remains in an unconscious state, and as long as his energy flows freely so that the I AM can express itself completely, the child is one with God, and dwells in the Garden of Eden, but once the child experiences his own separate identity, their total union is shattered and he is expelled from the garden and from his infantile state of bliss. It is from this moment, the moment of separation, that fear begins. With fear comes the "other," and the unconscious awareness that separation, living outside the ALL means extinction.

Rather than racing back to union, a child normally does the exact opposite. He begins to identify exclusively with his conscious self which dominates the ego and seeks to extinguish any remembrance of the unconscious innocence and bliss that once was. The conscious self then attempts to usurp the position of the I AM by glorifying itself and the state of duality in which it finds itself. It goes as far as denying the existence of anything else but duality. As a result, the child leaves innocence behind and by doing so begins living a life of striving where actions spring primarily from consciousness.

When a person's actions spring primarily from consciousness, his actions don't resonate from deep within them, from the center of his being and there is no deep sense of purpose in them, because they are not deeply rooted in the I AM. Contentment and security are lost, and as a result actions are performed out of desire and fear. Action then becomes striving after things which a person wants which either dull the pain, or help him avoid it.

The mere existence of the I AM intensifies the pain by constantly reminding a person of their fragmentation and superficiality; therefore it is a constant threat to consciousness and its position. Consciousness uses whatever weapon is available to it to defend itself against the I AM. It will do anything to retain its position.

In the parable of the servants we have the perfect metaphor of the bitter struggle:

33   There was certain householder (I AM) which planted a vineyard in it and hedged it roundabout and digged a winepress in it and built a tower and let it out to husbandman consciousness and went into a far country.

34   And when the time of the fruit drew near, he sent his servants to the husbandman, that

they might receive fruits of it.

35 And the husbandman took his servants, and beat one, and killed another and stoned another.

36 Again, he sent other servants more than the first, and they did unto them likewise.

37 But last of all he sent unto them his son saying, they will reverence my son.

38 But when the husbandmen saw the son, they said among themselves: This is the heir, come let us kill him and let us seize on his inheritance.

39 And they caught him, and cast him out of the vineyard and slew him.[11]

To transcend a life in which the ego is rooted primarily in consciousness and to achieve a true "self" centered wholeness, a person must confront fear, the fear of the unloved "others." Through the work of psychospiritual integration, the little demons imprisoned within the consciousness can be released and integrated. The work begins when a person confronts his fear and then is honest and courageous enough to admit that these demons exist. With courage, a person can accept them and recollect them. From recollection, a person can embrace them, integrating them with the rest of his "selves," and this reunion makes a person again childlike and brings him into a state of wholeness and unconditional joy.

CHAPTER VIII

TO THINE OWN "SELF" BE TRUE

Shall we perhaps, in purgatory, see our own
faces and hear our own voices as they really
are.

—C. S. Lewis
Reflections on the Psalms

Prerequisites

A person can only succeed in the work of psychospiritual
integration by approaching the work honestly and courageously. Honesty is the willingness to see things as they
truly are, not as you would like them to be. Courage is the
willingness to accept what you see. I have discovered
through my work that being honest and courageous can be
quite difficult for most people. The rules and conventions
of our society, the desire not to hurt other people's feelings,
the desire to be accepted, and the unconscious need to see
things as better or worse than they are, all conspire to make
a person fearful and dishonest.

There are many reasons why people have chosen to be
dishonest rather than honest. Sometimes dishonesty is the
easier choice—particularly in a situation that threatens
what a person perceives to be his security or well-being. In
this case, consciousness, in order to preserve things as they

are, decides that it is wiser to be dishonest. But more often people are dishonest with themselves and others to keep from experiencing more energy than they can handle. Although objectively having more energy is desirable because energy is the essential ingredient in good physical health, good relationship and the experience of unconditional joy, many people are aware that by becoming too healthy and too joyful, their life, work and one's network of relationships will be threatened. The condition of a person's life, the quality of his relationships, his personal strength, work and health are determined by his energy level and his ability to radiate all forms of energy freely. Each person's life is in effect a rationalization constructed to support the limits he has put on his personal energy flow. By changing the level of energy and the extent it can radiate, a person changes his relationship to the world. (A person's outer condition is always a reflection of his inner condition.) Any increase to a person's energy level, like Tagore said, can be threatening to a person who is "ever building this wall around." For this reason when asked to make a choice between honesty and more energy, or dishonesty and the status quo, most people will choose the status quo.

Blocking The Flow

Most people choose dishonesty, in particular emotional dishonesty, in order to block unwanted emotional energy from flowing through their subtle energy system. However, if a person lies to himself or to someone else about his feelings to avoid feeling something, he blocks the flow of energy and by doing so he disrupts his relationship. This can be either a partial or complete disruption, depending on circumstances. The point in the subtle energy system and the corresponding area of the physical body where a person becomes blocked depends on what frequencies of energy are being blocked. The net result, however, is that when the free radiation of energy is restricted, people feel less connected to each other.

The degree of separation experienced by both parties depends on the energy expended by the dishonest person to cover up their true feelings and how effective the cover-up is. Since few lies are truly effective, only a partial cover-up is usually accomplished and energy is restricted rather than completely blocked. By being only partially blocked, the energy will have its frequency distorted and this will disrupt the relationship. Moreover, by being dishonest, a person not only blocks energy radiating outward but he also blocks the free flow of energy within his own subtle energy system. If the coverup is continued over a length of time, the level of Prana within his subtle energy system will fall sharply.

Restricting the flow of Prana and covering up the truth is a continuous job. A person must continually work at it and expend a great deal of energy to successfully be dishonest. Notwithstanding all this work, it serves no useful purpose to be dishonest. All it does is disrupt relationships and cause unnecessary pain and suffering.

Thoughts and Emotions

Every thought and emotion is a radiation of energy generated by a subfield within a person's personal energy field. It is a property of energy to have motion, not to be static. Thoughts and emotions generated by a person's mental and astral (emotional) field are not only experienced by the mental and astral body generating the thoughts and emotions, but the thoughts and emotions radiate in all directions. They may begin by being localized in their own concentrations of mental and astral energy, but once the thoughts and emotions become manifest, they cannot be kept within their own localization. By the very nature of the universal field and its localizations, the mental and emotional energy radiates equally in all directions within its specific vibratory range. The broadcast of mental and emotional energy, like a broadcast of radio waves, will be picked up by any other localization tuned into or sensitive to its particular rate of vibration.

The energy created by thought and emotion or even animal magnetism which radiates from someone will affect every person in their immediate environment who is sensitive to the particular frequency being broadcast, or at a distance, if the thought or emotion is focused to a particular person. The radiations of mental and emotional energy which we are all subjected to are meant to nourish us. However, if we are caught in a distorted energy field caused by either emotional or mental dishonesty, our energy system will be disrupted and we will suffer a loss of energy as well as disruption in our ability to radiate freely.

The effect that thoughts and emotions have can be likened to waves created when a stone has been thrown into a still lake: the stone makes an impact at a certain point, and this impact radiates equally in all directions in a series of waves which make an impression on all objects within *its* medium or field. The impression will continue affecting the objects by causing a sympathetic vibration in their energy field until its effect is diluted by other waves within the medium. The amplitude of the wave depends on the size of the stone and the force of its delivery.

In the same way, the impact one person will have on another person is determined by the power and quality of the sender's thoughts and emotions, and receptivity of the receiver. This goes a long way in explaining the subtle dynamics of human interaction, the dynamics of trust and distrust, alienation, friendship and animosity, or the hypnotic effect one person can have on another or even on large groups. Moreover, it explains why as individuals we are often deeply affected both positively and negatively by people to whom we have no close ties or common interests.

Atmospheres

Thoughts and emotions which are confined to enclosed spaces such as homes and workplaces will have a particularly strong effect on people entering the space. Thoughts and emotions generated by an individual or group can remain in an enclosed space and can be absorbed by physical matter within it. The "atmosphere" of a room created in this way can linger long after the people who created the atmosphere or the feelings and thoughts have changed.

An individual will be affected by the "atmosphere" which has been created in this way, and will be affected positively or negatively depending on the quality of the atmosphere. This explains how moods can change so rapidly when a person simply moves from one room to another or one environment to another. An understanding of how the atmosphere of a room can influence people is important, because to become proficient in the use of energy, a person must understand the dynamics of energy in both healthy environments and disturbed environments caused by dishonesty.

Where the atmosphere is confined to small rooms, it is usually clearly discernible. Such is the case in many old and small chapels where the devotional feelings of thousands of people have literally charged the emotional and mental atmosphere of the room. Both the emotional and mental atmospheres in an enclosed space can create a wholesome nourishing environment or an unwholesome disruptive one. We are all subject to the influence of emotional and mental atmospheres, and a person should exercise caution before voluntarily submitting himself to those environments which clearly have a negative atmosphere and will have a negative influence on his energy system and on his general well-being.

Experiencing Atmospheres

The exercise below is designed to help you experience atmospheres more consciously. Once you try the exercise you will see that you are more sensitive to the mental and emotional atmospheres in a room and more influenced by them than you would have imagined. This is a group exercise and it works best with about five or six people. Each person will have one or two turns to experience the combined mental and emotional atmosphere that has been created by a group of people. A small meeting room would be best for this exercise, but a small office or living room will suffice. If you are a group of six people, begin by having each person choose a number from one to six that will determine which turn is theirs. Number one will be the first person to leave the room. The person who leaves the room will be called the "sensitive." The sensitive must go to a room where the words or even the voices of the people who are participating in the exercise cannot be heard. While the sensitive is outside, s/he should relax with eyes closed and activate his/her second attention.

People are remarkably sensitive to atmospheres, especially when they are experiencing the world through the second attention. While each person is outside of the room, the rest of the group should pick a topic which you all have strong feelings and ideas about, and for about five minutes you should engage each other in a lively discussion. Try to get to a dominant feeling like joy, fear or anger which you all share. For example you can talk about politics, ecology, friendship, love, death, children, etc. During the discussion each person should feel free to express their feelings and thoughts. Try to stay on one main theme for five minutes, and each person should remain consistent so that the atmosphere of the room becomes charged with strong, clearly defined feelings and ideas about the issue you are talking about.

After five minutes one of the group who has for their turn been designated leader should abruptly end the conversation and collect the missing member of the group. As soon as the sensitive enters the room, s/he should immediately begin telling the group about the changes s/he feels in the room.

On the mental level the sensitive might experience his/her mind being flooded by the thoughts which still linger in the room. These thoughts can come in verbal form or in pictures. On the emotional level s/he might feel the dominant mood or feeling of the group; or the emotions of the dominant members of the group. Or s/he might simply feel a vague atmosphere of excitement, warmth, anxiety, or depression.

If the sensitive is particularly receptive, s/he may discern the general topic of conversation and the views of dominant members of the group. His/her physical body will also register changes in the atmosphere. Anxiety will often be experienced as tightness in different parts of the sensitive's body. The body might become excited physically or even suddenly tired or lethargic. There are literally scores of different sensations which the sensitive's physical body will register. A person without training will miss many subtle vibrations since they are experienced on a barely conscious level. However, the dominant expressions of the group can easily be recognized by anyone. The sensitive must simply pay attention to the changes that are felt physically, emotionally and mentally upon entering the room.

After a full disclosure by both the sensitive and the group, you can proceed by sending the next person out and beginning again with a new topic of discussion. The old atmosphere will be dissipated once you start discussing your new topic. Keep repeating the exercise until everyone has at least one chance to be the sensitive.

Self-Improvement

Before we can completely understand the importance of being honest in a human relationship, we must have a working definition of honesty. Langenscheidt defines honesty as "trustworthy; not likely to lie or to cheat . . . not hiding the facts . . ."[1]

I can't argue with this definition, but I would go a bit farther and add that honesty is the complete, uncensored expression of a person's complex nature in every situation on all levels of causation with everyone with whom s/he is in relationship. Defined in this way, you can readily see that society has taught us that normal human interaction would be impossible if everyone was honest on all levels all the time.

The hypothesis from which this rationalization for dishonesty comes implies that we are inherently imperfect and our motives are impure, that our real feelings and thoughts are not good enough and have to be improved. It implies that we are defective, that unlike other species which fit into the ecology of this planet perfectly, we don't, and therefore we must make corrections in God's imperfect handiwork.

Society as we know it has suffered a severe setback in human development because of this belief. Its acceptance has caused a breakdown in honesty and trust, especially self-trust. Of course, some people in society claim to trust in someone or something, but this is not the trust I'm talking about.

The trust I'm talking about is the childlike trust which is derived from an inherent feeling of safety. It is a trust which is not only conscious, but is unconscious. It is a trust which underlies every thought, emotion and action. When trust in one's self and the world is missing, there can be no inherent honesty, because expressing yourself honestly requires having trust in one's self.

Belief Systems

A person who lacks trust will be prevented from achieving his personal goal of wholeness and unconditional joy. Moreover, a person who lacks trust must continuously block the feelings of emptiness and despair imprisoned within him from rising to the surface. As a consequence, he blocks his energy from radiating freely and the I AM from expressing itself.

In the place of the guidance of the I AM, he must substitute beliefs to guide his behavior. Those beliefs are nothing more than transparent substitutes for the intuitive guidance of the I AM. A belief system is formed through the interaction of a person's desires and fears. For better or worse, belief systems imprison the union of selves. In this regard the great French philosopher Rousseau wrote, "Man is born free, but everywhere he is in chains,"[2] and Jean de la Fontaine echoed this by saying, "What's the use of the good life, if you are not free?"[3]

For the vast majority of people, it is not the I AM radiating through the unconscious which determines how they will act, instead this most important power has been handed over to consciousness which acts according to the rules laid down by the person's belief system.

Consciousness uses the ego to police the inner levels of awareness, and it does its job with blind fanaticism. It will keep a person in line by forcing him to obey the rules which form the basis of his belief system. It uses fear to intimidate and pain to punish. In this condition a person is not permitted to question the legitimacy of these rules. He is simply required to obey them. It doesn't matter where the rules come from. It doesn't matter that for the most part they are simply a collection of old baggage: thoughts and feelings which were handed down from family, school and society. It doesn't matter that they don't truly reflect the person's deepest aspirations and needs, that they are the product of fear and desire, that they aren't rooted in the I AM but instead are the product of insecurity which results from a lack of self-trust. All that matters is that the I AM remains imprisoned and that consciousness remains secure in its position.

The Fruits of Dishonesty

The result of living dishonestly is that although each person seeks to protect others, maintain good relationships and create a just and happy society, the methods he has chosen to accomplish these goals simply don't work. More importantly, the methods employed institutionalize the injustice, isolation and pain we see everywhere around us. For all our efforts we have come no closer to personal or national harmony than our ancestors came in the past. And so in an effort not to fall into a state of hopelessness and despair, most people hope for a future where someone else might put a bandage on their bleeding wounds. But hope in the future is part of the game. Hope too, is based on fear.

"L'esperance et la crainte sont inseparables, et il n'y a point de crainte sans esperance, ni d'esperance sans crainte." (Hope and fear are inseparable; you cannot have fear without hope and you cannot have hope without fear.)[4]

It is not surprising to anyone who has studied human nature that by restricting their unconscious life and the natural expression of the I AM, a person must suffer severe consequences.

The avoidance of the inner life because of fear, and its offspring dishonesty, is at the root of the individual's and society's problems. Whatever is blocked and repressed within a person, whatever is not allowed its free expression and experienced within must be sought outside in the external world, and if it is not found outside himself a person will substitute some distorted desire or goal for it.

Self-Indulgence

By substituting a distorted desire or goal for the unconditional joy offered by the I AM, a person falls into the bottomless pit of self-indulgence. The institutions of society are partly to blame, because instead of producing self-possessed people who experience unconditional joy within themselves, society has turned out people who are dishonest and afraid, who forever seek comfort from someone or something outside themselves. Because of this, people have become confused. They have become riddled by conflict and ambivalence. Most people have lost sight of where they are going. They have lost their way. They are hearing so many voices that the intuitive voice of the I AM is almost totally obscured. Unreal goals have been substituted for real ones, unreal needs for real ones, and unreal desires for real ones. And so each individual and mankind in general rushes madly into the future searching for a peace and contentment they cannot possibly find because they search for it outside themselves.

Self-indulgence is the alternative chosen by those who have lost access to the I AM. It takes the form of all sorts of addictive behavior, from overeating to excessive worrying, self-importance, arrogance to depression, alcoholism and even drug addiction and suicide. You indulge yourself when you are not being yourself, and you are driven to self-indulgence by the pain of being fragmented rather than integrated. It is by being honest that one begins the work of psychospiritual integration. By choosing honesty, a person can remember himself (his unconscious selves), recollect them and integrate them with his conscious self. From that point, energy work becomes easy. It becomes the unconscious harmonious working of spirit, soul and body. From the Tao we read: " . . . in the pursuit of the way (the self) one does less every day. One does less and less until one does nothing at all. And one does nothing at all, there is nothing that is left undone . . . "[5]

The story below illustrates the need for honesty in the work of psychospiritual integration.

A prominent Sufi of Central Asia was examining young men who wanted to become his disciples. He asked them: "Is there anyone here who wants entertainment rather than learning, who wishes to argue not study, who is impatient, who wants to take rather than to give? If there is, he should raise his hand." Nobody moved. "Very good" said the teacher, "now you will come and see some of my pupils, who have been with me for three years." He led them into a meditation hall, where a row of people were sitting. Addressing them, he said: "Let those who wish to be entertained, rather than learn, and want to argue not study, those who are impatient, who would rather take than give—let them stand up." The whole row of disciples got to their feet. The sage addressed the first group. "In your own eyes you are better people now than you could be in three years' time if you stayed here. Your present vanity (dishonesty) helps you feel more worthy than these students who for three years have selflessly devoted themselves to the work. So reflect well, as you return to your homes, before coming here again at some future time if you wish, whether you want to feel better than you are."[6]

Courage

It takes courage to choose honesty in the face of fear. And it is courage which is the second prerequisite for the work of psychospiritual integration. When I say courage I don't mean physical courage alone, or the heroism we see in extraordinary circumstances or crisis. I mean the everyday courage which gives life its nobility, which gives a person the strength to choose himself over what other people want him to be; I mean the courage which enables a person to trust himself and have the honesty to be himself in every situation so that he can live his own life and follow his own Dharma. When I say courage, I mean the courage in little things which says yes to "self," yes to life, which is life-affirming.

In Hermetics we learn that "everything is dual, everything has poles, everything has its pair of opposites."[7] Life consists of the balance of opposites, it rests in the midst of this duality. We can say that we have life because of this duality and without it, life would not be possible. As a consequence, life must consist of fear and courage, and by existing within this balance, life resists the inertia toward extinction. Courage does not overcome or erase fear. Courage is the process of taking fear into itself. It is the antithesis of avoidance and self-indulgence. Courage is affirmation. It says yes to everything, it embraces everything, even the possibility of one's own extinction. By embracing the possibility of extinction, non-being, it accepts the ultimate terrifying possibility and continues to radiate in spite of the possibility of non-being. In a universe resting in duality there is "being" only because there is "non-being."[8]

"Courage is the power of life to affirm itself . . . while the negation of life (despair) because of its negativity is an expression of cowardice." Paul Tillich tells us that courage which says yes to self and is self-affirming" . . . is the essential nature of every being and as such its highest good. Perfect self-affirmation is not an isolated act which originates in the individual being, but is participation in the universal or divine act of self-affirmation, which is the originating power in every individual act.[9]

" . . . He hath heart who knoweth fear but vanquishes it, who seeth the abyss, but with pride. He who seeth the abyss (non-being) but with eagle's talons graspeth the abyss; he hath courage."[10]

To understand courage is to understand that the lack of

it is not the only problem. Another problem in dealing with the courage is ambivalence. It is misplaced courage caused by the split between what the I AM perceives as good and desirable, what it chooses as its goals and defends, what unconsciously the "others" caused by fragmentation perceive as good and desirable, and what they unconsciously choose as their goals and defend. The goals of success and happiness which promote the free radiation of energy will not be triumphant; they will not resonate from deep within a person if on the unconscious level a person has goals which are in opposition. On the unconscious level, the goals of the unloved "others" always revolve around recreating "particular feelings" which make a person feel safe and secure, close to a person whom they loved as a child. If a person has goals which are in opposition to these feelings, a person will have problems achieving them because his loyalty will be to the old feelings and he will defend them with great courage.

It does not matter if the old feelings are positive or negative. To reject the feelings a person must reject someone he loved as a child who left an imprint in his personal energy field. The imprints are these "particular feelings," and having these feelings as an adult allows a person to feel unconsciously that he is still in relationship with the beloved person. The courage of self-affirmation means releasing these feelings, processing the energy which the "unconscious others" are holding on to because you recognize that they are ultimately self-defeating since they oppose goals of freedom, love and success. This demands the rejection of any relationship based on the old feelings, as well. Giving up the old relationship and the particular feelings requires great courage because there is no guarantee that a relationship of any kind will be possible with the beloved, once the feelings are released. It is the fear of losing the treasured feelings and the relationship they symbolize which makes the courage to affirm self so difficult to achieve and at the same time so important. Instead of having the courage to defend a relationship which when in opposition to your goals of success and love becomes life defeating, a person must substitute the courage to do only what is life-affirming.

Freud said that a healthy person is one who can love and one who can work. Anything in your life, any feeling which gets in the way of either, must be looked at honestly and accepted, and then you must have the courage to release it and say goodbye to it.

You need to care enough for yourself to accept and then release the old self-destructive feelings which you have so courageously defended for so many years. Courage is intuitively connected to caring for your self. This deep caring involves the sacrifice of something you once treasured for something greater, that being personal freedom and unconditional joy. A person must be willing to give up all his pearls for the great pearl, himself.

The act of sacrifice takes great courage because it is in one sense like death. Thomas Merton, the great theologian, tells us "in order to realize himself, man has to risk the diminuition and even the total loss of all his reality in favor of another, for if any man would have his life, he must lose it."[11]

CHAPTER IX

BECOMING FEARLESS

Mein Geist durstet nach Taten, mein Atem nach freiheit.

> —Schiller

Disrupting Fear

The principle manifestation of fear is contraction. On the physical level this reflex can be useful, as when a child learns that fire hurts by putting his finger too close to a candle or by touching a hot pan. But beyond this physical response it has little instructive value. Da Free John tells us:[1]

"Fear is just an ordinary mechanism that you master . . . It has no ultimate philosophical significance."

Because of the destructive nature of fear and anxiety, especially prolonged fear which can become addictive and pervasive, I have included several techniques in this chapter designed to transmute and release fear. The first technique was developed by the ancient yogis. It is a breathing technique, based on the way infants breathe. It is called the Yogic Breath. It is a completely natural form of breathing. It is the way your body wants to breathe when it is at rest. By practicing it regularly, you can go a long way toward disrupting and dissipating the fear mechanism in your life.

The Yogic Breath

The Yogic Breath is a synthesis of three breaths, and it is often called the complete breath. It is always done through the nose, and there is no separation between inhalation and exhalation. You can begin practicing the Yogic Breath as a separate exercise or as part of your meditations and relaxation exercises. However, after a short time it should become your normal way of breathing. (You will probably notice that you are breathing yogically when the second attention is active.) The Yogic Breath will always accompany a deep state of relaxation, and a person breathes yogically when there is a healthy balance between consciousness and unconsciousness.

There are three parts to the Yogic Breath. The first is the abdominal breath. In the abdominal breath the abdomen is expanded and stretched downward as you breathe in; the second part is the mid-breath. In the mid-breath the air, once having filled the abdomen, expands to fill the chest cavity, expanding the rib cage and lifting the shoulders. The third and last part is the nasal breath. In the nasal breath the air, having first filled the abdomen and then the chest, fills the throat and nose and continues filling the nasal passages.

To use this technique to transmute fear into a healthy state of relaxation and peace, follow the instructions below:

Begin by sitting in a comfortable position with your back straight and your legs flat on the floor. You can use the lotus position if you like. Once you're sitting comfortably, place your right hand on your abdomen just below the solar plexus. This will help you feel the rhythm of your breath and will make it more fluid. Then close your eyes. Closing the eyes is not essential but it will help you to relax, making yogic breathing easier. Begin by breathing in, first filling your lower lungs with air. With your hand on your abdomen, you will feel the muscles of your diaphragm stretch as your stomach becomes slightly extended. Continue breathing inward, feeling the air fill the middle and upper part of your lungs. Your shoulders will lift and the muscles of the rib cage will stretch as the lungs expand. During the mid-breath, some people feel pain in the upper back between the shoulder blades. The pain is caused by muscles which over the years have contracted and have become stiff. This is largely due to improper breathing. Don't let a little discomfort discourage you, press on. In a few days the discomfort will disappear and your muscles will return to their normal state of elasticity.

After air has filled your lungs, let it continue to rise, filling your nasal passages and head, giving you a light, pleasant sensation. When you exhale, reverse the process, letting the nasal passages empty first, then the upper, mid and finally the lower lungs. Your shoulders will naturally drop and the diaphragm will then return to its normal position. Without separation between inhalation and exhalation, continue this exercise for about five minutes.

At first, reserve special times during the day for practice, but once the rhythm is mastered, make this form of breathing the norm. Become attentive to your breathing and gently bring it back to the complete breath every time it becomes shallow or falls into an old habit. Now, *a note of warning:* be sure that you are gentle with yourself. Don't fall victim to watching yourself and your breathing all the time. Don't become obsessive about it, because you will simply cause yourself unnecessary anxiety, and instead of helping yourself to radiate more freely you will restrict yourself even more.

Gross Effects

Yogic breathing is useful in disrupting the reflex of fear because it prevents a person from contracting and blocking the flow of energy through one's subtle energy system. By holding the breath between inhalation and exhalation and by taking shallow breaths, feelings are restricted and effectively deadened. That's why people tend to hold their breath and don't breathe deeply during times of stress.

The use of breathing exercises to help a person calm down and reduce the impact of stress has become widely accepted by both the medical community and more recently by the business community. Dr. Phillip Nuernberger, who serves as a stress-management consultant for corporations, has run several tests on the use of breathing techniques for relaxation. In one experiment he taught a group yogic breathing techniques and used another group as a control. When breathing yogically, the trained group consistently scored better on standard psychological tests and lower on the so-called neuroticism scale than the group who did not breathe yogically.

Furthermore, in two independent studies from the University of California, J. V. Hardt and B. Timmons proved that there is a link between breathing and the quality of brain waves. They found more alpha waves, which are known to appear when people are relaxed, during deep breathing, and they found fewer when people were engaged in fast, shallow breathing. The alpha waves correlated better when breathing was deep, full and rhythmic than when it was shallow and less rhythmic.

Even in people who breathe shallowly and arhythmically, the body can automatically release fear and tension by releasing the breath in the form of a sigh, or groan. This instinctive reaction points to the possibility of using the body's unconscious mechanisms for processing large doses of stress or anxiety. Using this unconscious mechanism as a starting point, we go one step further and use tone and vibration in place of a sigh or groan to consciously transmute fear and its characteristic contraction. The technique is called "resonating."

Resonating

Resonating can be practiced almost anywhere you can make audible sounds without being disturbed or disturbing someone else. Resonating will go a long way in reducing the negative effects of anxiety due to prolonged stress. You can begin practicing the technique by finding a comfortable position with your back straight. Once you are comfortable, begin breathing yogically. After about two minutes bring your mental attention to your heart, and instead of breathing yogically initiate each breath from your heart until you feel deep feelings resonating from it. On each inhalation, feel the emotion in your heart growing stronger. And on each exhalation, surrender to the feeling and allow it to radiate through your chest and from there through your whole body.

Feel the energy coming from your heart, radiating through your arms, legs, stomach, sexual organs, head, skin, etc. Exhale without a break in the rhythm of your breathing. After about two minutes of breathing in this way, place the tip of your tongue to the top of your palate just behind your teeth and put your hands together in front of you. Then on each exhalation as you feel the emotions of your heart beginning to radiate, put sound to the feeling and chant *ohm* for the full duration of your exhalation.*

Feel the sound you chant emanating from deep within your heart and let it resonate so that your whole body vibrates from it. Let it become the singular expression of what you are experiencing and feeling. It is not necessary to chant too loudly, but it is best when you chant audibly. Continue chanting for about five minutes. The effects of the exercise, especially after you have been doing it for a few days or weeks, are profound. Not only does the technique transmute fear, it replaces fear with feelings of well-being

---

* Ohm in Sanskrit is the sound of the universal vibration. This is the sound uttered by the All at the moment of creation. It is the combined sound of all created things.

and contentment. This exercise is particularly helpful in developing the second attention since it opens the heart and at the same time quiets the mind and brings you into a state of full body consciousness.

Resonating should be practiced regularly during times of prolonged stress or anxiety. It will have a continuous rejuvenating effect. Used as a regular exercise it will disrupt fear in the form of anxiety, self-doubt, insecurity, confusion, alienation and worry. I recommend that you include this exercise in your daily regimen. Practice it in the morning before breakfast and just before going to bed. It is particularly helpful for people who have trouble falling asleep because of excessive anxiety or worry.

Subtle Effects

By resonating and breathing yogically you will free yourself from the gross effects of fear, and you will begin to experience changes physically, emotionally, and mentally. Your physical body will feel more relaxed, your emotions will be more under control and your mind will become clearer and quieter. Energy supports these effects. Through correct breathing and resonating, more Prana is circulated through the subtle energy system, and this has a beneficial effect on all levels. On the mental level, proper breathing will lower brain-wave frequency and as a result the "internal dialogue" (the internal dialogue is the excessive mental chatter which endlessly disrupts most people's peace of mind) will be disrupted. By having the brain wave frequency lowered, the brain will begin to operate more efficiently and it will substitute visual thought for verbal thought. Lower brain-wave frequency also permits the unconsciousness to become more active, creating a healthier balance between consciousness and unconsciousness. This balance permits a person to operate throughout his entire mental range.

An increase in Prana also permits a person to feel expansive and open by freeing reservoirs of emotional energy trapped by fear. Increases in Prana can be experienced in many ways, some of which can feel odd at first. Some people get hot throughout the whole body when the flow of Prana is increased, and some people feel heat, particularly in the hands and/or feet. Most people feel vibrations and tingling sensations. There is no danger in these sensations. However, if your hands become numb or cramped, it means that you have been hyperventilating. To counteract this, immediately stop deep breathing. If someone is with you, have him take your hands in his. If you are alone, put your hands together, put your tongue on the roof of your mouth behind your teeth and breathe normally. In a short time your body will feel fine.

Many people feel lightheaded or slightly dizzy when they breathe yogically or resonate. This is normally experienced by beginners who have a low energy level and who aren't used to higher levels of Prana in the subtle energy system. It is not something to be concerned about, since it rarely goes on for any length of time.

As the energy system gets used to channeling more Prana, these side-effects will go away. By freeing the flow of Prana, people normally feel more open emotionally. Sometimes by breathing yogically or resonating people feel sadness, joy, even compassion coming up. Breathing yogically and resonating have the tendency to disrupt energy blockages. It is not uncommon to have old feelings coming to the surface. If they do come up, let them flow through your energy system and allow your energy system to release them.

While practicing yogic breathing or resonating, your heart might begin to beat quickly. This is normally a temporary reaction and you shouldn't be alarmed by it. There is also the possibility that you will experience pain at some point in your physical body where energy has been blocked. These physical blockages correspond to blockages in the astral and mental bodies. Most often these pains are experienced at the points where the chakras are located. Pains such as these are rarely severe and rarely persist after you complete your breathing exercises. However, they can go on for several weeks during exercises until the area has been opened and more Prana is permitted to flow through it.

In the East, for centuries adepts have freed themselves from the limitations imposed by fear by breathing yogically, resonating and studying Pranayama, the science of breath. Moreover, they have learned to increase their physical, emotional, mental and spiritual well-being by practicing breathing exercises regularly. Over the centuries the adepts have learned that "One can bring himself into a harmonious vibration with nature and aid in the unfoldment of his latent powers . . . by controlled breathing he may not only cure disease in himself and others, but also practically do away with fear and worrying . . . "[2]

Is Stress the Enemy

Inordinate fear and shock can overload the subtle energy system. Shock is usually a sudden, unexpected experience which forces the subtle energy system to process an excessive amount of Prana almost instantaneously. If there are blockages in a person's subtle energy system, instantaneous processing is almost impossible. When a person is unable to process all the energy flowing through him, the unprocessed part is trapped in the system and forms "reservoirs." These reservoirs can have a serious and longterm effect on a person.

A typical situation which can overload the subtle energy energy system occurs as you're driving on the freeway or expressway. You're relaxed, listening to the radio for example, and suddenly without warning the car slightly ahead of you jumps into your lane. You jam your foot down on the brake and manage to avoid hitting the car. But that's not the end of it. Although you've avoided an accident, your heart pounds, your hands feel hot and sweaty and you feel sick to your stomach.

This is a typical stress/shock reaction common to all human beings. However, the nausea that a person experiences is not from the shock itself but from the fact that the person did not process all the energy shooting through the subtle energy system. As a result, the physical body was unable to release and properly distribute the valuable chemical byproducts of that shock/stess response.

At the moment of shock, the physical body delivers adrenalin, blood sugar, cortisone and ACTH into the system. But the package must be delivered to the appropriate destination. Energy is the carrier. If energy is blocked, the physical chemicals are also blocked and they get stuck in places they don't belong. If the package fails to reach the appropriate destination soon enough, it will end up in the pit of your stomach and it will make you feel sick and nauseous. To avoid this painful situation as well as to avoid creating unwanted reservoirs of Prana, the next time you are in a shocking situation use the technique below to prevent overload:

The moment you are first shocked, open your mouth and scream as loudly as you can. At the same time pull your arms into your sides as hard as you can. Tense your legs, chest, arms (as many areas of your body as you can as quickly as possible); keep up the tension as long as you can because this will permit the package of energy and chemicals to be distributed through your Nadis (energy channels) and to your tense muscles. Once you feel relieved and you feel energy flowing normally through your body, you can relax.

It's interesting to note that your body does not know

the difference between sudden fear and sudden anger. It delivers the same package of energy and chemicals in either case.

If you have ever been in a situation where you were subjected to a tongue lashing that you felt was completely unwarranted, and you stood there and took it without visibly reacting, you now understand why you felt emotionally blocked and sick to your stomach after it was over. Your subtle energy system and your physical body reacted but consciously you didn't. As a result, the package of energy and chemicals didn't go where they were supposed to.

To keep this from happening again, as soon as you feel sudden anger or any excessive emotion for that matter and you can't scream, put your hands behind your back and repeat the last exercise, except instead of screaming out loud, forcibly push the air out of your mouth so that you can hear it. Then pull the air back in through your nose. Repeat a second time in the same way. Continue until you feel energy radiating through your body in all directions and you feel a lightness in your body and head. When you finish the technique, instead of feeling horrible you will feel relaxed and absolutely wonderful (particularly when you realize how much good you've done for yourself energetically and physically).

To understand the basic mechanism at work in both the sudden fear and sudden anger situation, you must realize that your nervous system and subtle energy system are at the minimum several million years old. They were designed to react instantaneously to life-threatening situations. In a situation that was threatening, your autonomic (or automatic) nervous system as well as your subtle energy system delivered a package of energy and chemicals to give you an added boost whether you stood and fought or ran for the nearest tree. If you were going to stand and fight, the package poured into your arm and chest muscles and gave you short-term superhuman strength.

All of you have heard or read of cases where slightly built people responded to a crisis situation with sudden and incredible strength. Now you know where the energy came from. The burst of energy you receive in a threatening situation is designed to help you, not harm you. However, you must be able to process it so that your subtle energy system and physical body are not overloaded. Practice the exercises in this chapter, and in the future you will be free from the negative effect or fear and overload, and you will have far more health-giving energy at your disposal.

CHAPTER X

THE PHYSICAL BODY

Aum,—may all the parts of my body,
my eyes, ears, speech and life, all the strength
of my senses get nourishment in Him.
All beings are actually Brahma . . .
—*The Upanishads*

Central to the work of psychospiritual integration is the
concept that the physical body is the outward manifestation
of a series of subtler bodies. These subtler bodies, together
with the energy of the physical body, make up a person's
personal energy field. The subtle bodies interpenetrate
each other as well as the physical body which clothes them.
They are held together by the magnetic force of the universal field which not only interpenetrates them, but surrounds them as well and connects them to it. Most, if not all
the spiritual, philosophical and psychological teachings
and writings that have appeared and remain extant today,
bear witness to this concept. It is central to Tantric, Taoist,
Jungian and Yogic teachings. These systems, as well as the
Western metaphysical tradition, teach that each human
being is a reflection of the entire universe. If we can understand how we function as individuals we can understand
how the macrocosm functions, and if we can integrate our

"selves" and become whole by experiencing the I AM, the union of "selves," we can also experience the "All" as it radiates through the I AM. In this way we can experience union with the universal field.

But to understand ourselves as multidimensional beings, as a synthesis of subtle as well as physical bodies, we must understand the physical body in its true ecology, in its relationship to its subtle counterparts and the universal field. The physical body is the I AM's point of contact with the physical world.

The physical body which is made of dense physical matter is polarized negatively. It is receptive and therefore by nature Yin, fundamentally feminine. This is in accordance with the hermetic principle of gender which states that "gender is in everything: everything has its masculine and feminine principles; gender manifests on all planes."[1] The physical body that clothes the subtler bodies has an esoteric significance which goes beyond its obvious physical functions. In his first letter to the Corinthians, the Apostle Paul tells them "Know ye not that ye are the temple of God, and that the spirit of God dwelleth in you."[2]

It is the physical body, much like the temple of Jerusalem, which covers and in some ways protects the subtle bodies of man. This idea of the physical body being the temple of the spirit, as well as being the physical counterpart of a series of subtler bodies composed of matter of finer vibrations, is reflected in many lands by the layout and design of places of worship. The layout of churches and cathedrals in Europe reflect this idea. They are laid out in the shape of a cross which is the shape of a man lying down with his hands stretched out. This basic design is found also in Hebrew sanctuaries as well as temples in ancient Egypt and India.

The physical body which covers the I AM—the union of "selves"—is considered sacred in many traditions, and believers are admonished to treat the physical body with deference and not to defile it. There is intuitive wisdom in these admonitions, since the physical body has direct contact with the subtler bodies and can influence them.

Mistreatment of the physical body can and often does lead to disruption of the subtle energy system and the proper function of the higher bodies.

Victor Kulvinskas tells us:

> Mistreatment or accidents to the physical body also affect the etheric body since it must employ its energy to repair the physical body. If, due to mistreatment of the physical body, the etheric body is overworked, the etheric vitality is drained and the etheric body is unable to properly transmit impressions made by the mental and emotional bodies. The person in this condition seems to be mentally and emotionally unresponsive.

> It becomes clear that the physical body and the subtle bodies must all work together as a team. This can be accomplished when their vibratory rates are in proper alignment with each other just as the strings of a piano must be tuned so that the notes are in harmony with each other.[3]

Religious temples normally have three divisions: an outer courtyard, an innner court and a sacred shrine. The Hebrews call the sacred shrine the Holy of the Holies. This configuration reflects the esoteric partition of the human body which in the ancient teaching has three divisions. The outer courtyard of the temple where the uninitiated or lay population were allowed corresponds to the abdomen, pelvis and lower spine . . . this region contains the organs of digestion and reproduction. The significance energetically is that the student must attain a proper understanding of these functions as well as achieving their harmonious and balanced functioning before they are ready to move deeper into the temple and learn about more subtle teachings and energies

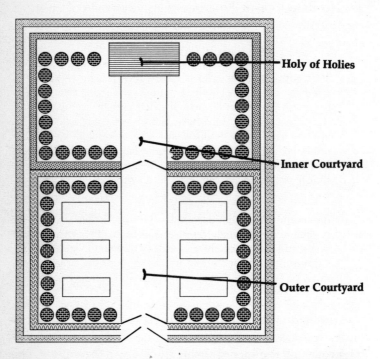

— Holy of Holies

— Inner Courtyard

— Outer Courtyard

Religious Temple as it corresponds to the three esoteric divisions of the human body.

contained within. In this phase they work consciously to achieve balance in the physical body as well as in the rational, conscious mind. In Yoga, the outer courtyard corresponds to Hatha, and in the Hebrew religion this conforms to the Mosaic law. In Japan, the abdomen has a further significance: it is believed to be the center of the physical body. Three fingers below the navel is the Hara. The word literally translated means belly, but to the Japanese it means more than that. It is the center, the point on which everything that we are, visible and invisible, is balanced. Graf von Durckheim described Hara as "nothing other than the physical embodiment of original life center in man."

In psychospiritual integration, the work a person must do while they remain in the outer courtyard corresponds to the preliminary work which the student must complete, which I call physical integration. While in the outer courtyard they develop courage and learn to express themself honestly. Through their conscious mind they learn about Dharma (life path) and bring the rational mind and physical body into a wholesome balance. Once they succeed in this work, they move from the outer courtyard to the inner courtyard, then the student is prepared to take the first step into the realm of higher consciousness and to begin the real work of psychospiritual integration. It is then that they enter the inner courtyard which corresponds to the area of the physical body lying between the neck and solar plexus.

The Internal Dialogue

The first obstacle to a student's progress—once they have crossed the threshold into the inner courtyard—is the internal dialogue.*

When the conscious mind is out of control, the subtler bodies remain imprisoned by this incessant mental chatter.

---

* The internal dialogue is the incessant mental chatter that goes on most of the time in people's minds.

The internal dialogue keeps a person cut off from a conscious experience of their subtle bodies and thus their inner life. Internal dialogue is a formidable obstacle to psychospiritual integration. The dervishes twirl and chant to dissipate it, students of Zen practice Za-Zen meditation in order to still the mind and suppress it; students of Yoga practice Pranayama to the same end.

I have developed a simple technique, a simple mental tool which will help you quiet the internal dialogue for a time so that you can function within the inner courtyard, activate the second attention and achieve mental balance.

In Zen, the state in which the internal dialogue has been eradicated is called no mind. Concerning this state, Ling-Chiao asks the Zen master Hui-Neng:

Q: I have left my home to become a monk and my aspiration is to attain Buddhahood. How should I use my mind?

A: Buddhahood is attained when there is no mind which is to be used for the task.

Q: When there is no mind to be used for the task, who can ever attain Buddhahood?

A: By no-mind the task is accomplished by itself. Buddha too has no mind.[4]

Beep Meditation

I call the technique for disrupting the internal dialogue the Beep meditation. It is a "not doing" exercise because rather than learning something new which will fill you up with more doing, it has the property of creating space . . . bringing you into a condition where you are not doing anything but where something can happen to you, where the I AM can emerge, the second attention can become active, and the internal dialogue can be extinguished.

Consciousness eternally seeks to control you and keep you in the outer courtyard. It does this by keeping you busy filling all your empty time with doing, feeling, acting and particularly by thinking. But none of this doing is deeply rooted, none of it resonates deeply through unconsciousness. By filling your time with doing, consciousness keeps you stranded on the surface in superficiality and as a result you never experience your "selves" in their fullness.

To experience the depths of your being, you must momentarily cut your exclusive attachment to consciousness by severing your attachment to thoughts which are generated from your conscious mind or enter your conscious mind from outside. This is where the Beep comes in. In the Beep meditation, every time a thought appears in your mind, you say "beep." Say it out loud; it is more effective that way. And don't struggle with the thought floating through your mind. You don't want to push it away (pushing is a form of doing and it gives additional power to the thought). You want the thought to dissipate, without it diverting your attention and affecting your emotions.

To begin the Beep meditation, find a comfortable position with your back straight and begin breathing deeply through your nose without separation between inhalation and exhalation. After a minute or two, or when you feel relaxed, mentally affirm "I am now deeply relaxed." Then let your mind drift to its perfect place of relaxation, what I call its "sanctuary." Your sanctuary is a place you create mentally. It is a place with no appointments to keep, no bills to pay, no stress to disturb you. It is a place where you feel content and free from anxiety, doubts, insecurities, etc., and where you are at peace with yourself and the environment around you. It doesn't matter whether it is somewhere on Earth or a place that you create on the mental plane. The important thing is that it becomes a place of complete rest (a place of renewal) for you. While you are there, enjoy yourself and relax completely. Remain in your sanctuary for about ten minutes. Stay awake and alert. Be attentive, let the second attention become active and experience your sanctuary as completely as you can.

After ten minutes mentally return to the room where you are meditating, take a deep breath and go deeper. Then begin paying attention to the thoughts that fill your mind, and each time a thought enters your mind say "beep." Stay relaxed when you say "beep." Don't say it with any emphasis or force. Remember, you are not pushing thoughts out of your mind. You are only detaching yourself from them and preventing your mind from consciously following any line of thought. This confuses your conscious mind, and in effect makes room for the unconscious mind to break through and flood the ego with its awareness. When the unconscious is given room and finds its rightful balance alongside consciousness, a person will experience the world through the second attention and directly experience the I AM. After some experience a person will be able to balance the second attention with the first attention, unconsciousness with consciousness, and in the course of any daily activity they will begin sensing energy fields which could be anything from atmospheres to personal energy fields or radiations from the universal field.

I want you to continue to beep thoughts out of your mind for about 20 minutes. In the beginning, the consciousness will balk at having its position threatened by fighting back with a barrage of thoughts, sometimes terribly negative ones. Don't be threatened or afraid. This is normal and is a sign of the conscious mind's weakness. Remember, fear is the only real weapon the consciousness has. The more thoughts the consciousness throws at you, the more you beep. After a little while (perhaps even in the first meditation) consciousness will get tired and accepts its fate, the I AM will emerge and you will experience some open space where there are no thoughts at all. After twenty minutes are up, mentally repeat this affirmation for about five minutes

"I am that I AM," and pay attention to how you feel physically, emotionally and mentally. You will notice that your mind is clear, you will feel light, full of energy, and you will have a full and deep sense of self-centered wholeness. I suggest you practice this exercise at least every other day, until you have control over the inner dialogue.

The Inner Courtyard

Once the internal dialogue is under control, the student will be firmly within the inner courtyard. The diaphragm symbolically divides the lower section, the abdomen (the outer courtyard) from the upper part of a person's esoteric anatomy. The upper section, the box formed by the rib cage, corresponds to the inner courtyard where initiates and priests, those who put their physical house (their physical body) and their conscious mind in order, are permitted to go. This chamber contains the heart, lungs, organs or respiration and the thymus, which by regulating the immunological system is the guardian of physical health. The diaphragm is said to separate the mundane physical world from the higher worlds of subtle vibrations. By ascending into the inner court the student has taken an important step in psychospiritual integration by moving from the gross physical plane to the subtle planes from the visual world to the non-visual world.

By moving beyond the diaphragm and entering the inner courtyard, the student begins in earnest the process of remembrance and recollection. By putting the physical house in order, a person begins to release the energy trapped by blockages in the first and second chakra, and the energy begins to move freely up to the solar plexus center. Once the student moves beyond the diaphragm, the energy trapped in the solar plexus and heart centers can be released. From the Upanishads we read "This God, the Great Soul, Creator of the Universe exists in the depth of the hearts of the people. With the well-cultivated reasoning, and the knowledge of mind, and the intuition of heart, He may be realized."[5]

In the Vedas, the heart is known as the seat of Brahma. It is often described as a lotus flower. Once the heart center is free to express itself, the student begins to experience the radiations from that center consciously. It is then that the flower begins to blossom with a bright green light. This light can be seen clearly by anyone with clairvoyant vision. Moreover, since the heart center is connected to the Ajna center (the third eye), by opening the heart center the student has access to the energy and awareness of the sixth chakra. Yogic tradition tells us that the Ajna center is the seat of our higher conscious self.

Having entered the inner court, the student begins to work on the higher planes . . . through the astral body (emotional body), they learn to transmute energy directly from the heart center to the Ajna center and they learn to conduct higher frequencies of Prana directly through the heart for use in healing. At this point the student begins to experience what the apostle Paul called the gifts of the spirit: wisdom, knowledge, faith, healing, miracles and prophecy. These gifts become accessible to the initiate when they have entered the inner court, because they now have access to the Ajna center through the heart.

The Holy of Holies

The Holy of Holies corresponds to the head where we find four organs of particular importance in psychospiritual integration: the brain, pituitary gland, pineal gland and tongue. The brain, the largest and most important organ in the head, governs the body in the same way that ultimately it is the "All" who governs the universe.

At the base of the brain is the pituitary gland. It was long believed by scientists and metaphysicians alike to be the center of spiritual perception. It is part of the endocrine system and can be considered to be the endocrine control center, since to some degree it exerts an influence over all other endocrines. In the past, several years' research has revealed important functions which relate to its significance in psychospiritual integration. In 1976, after years of study psychologists concluded that within the pituitary gland there are lengthy amino acids which after suitable transformation lead to the release of endorphins. Endorphins are natural pain killers found within the human body which are activated by stress or physical shock. Endorphine level has been linked to a person's pleasure level and to the experience of unconditional joy. One group of medical researchers hypothesize that laughter triggers the release of endorphins. Other research suggests that music, extended vigorous exercise such as jogging and the practice of Zen or Yogic meditations can stimulate the production of endorphins as well.

Located just behind the pituitary gland is the pineal gland. Like the pituitary gland, it is a ductless gland and is part of the endocrine system. It is cone shaped and about the size of a pea. There was some evidence that its function was connected to growth. Some medical authorities suggested that the gland affected sexuality, brain growth and the growth of intellect.

Recent research, however, links the pineal gland with altered states of consciousness and with the experience of transcendental union. Melatonin, a chemical found naturally in the brain and synthesized by the pineal gland, is an agent which naturally induces what previously were considered mystical states of consciousness. Melatonin is related to harmaline, a psychodelic drug processed from the Banisteriopsis vines of the Amazon and weakly linked to LSD. Harmaline has long been used by the Indians of the region to induce altered states of consciousness and psi experiences.

No wonder in so many tribal traditions the pineal gland was considered the seat of psi power and why so many ancient philosophers and scientists considered the pineal gland to be the seat of the soul. Alice Bailey, basing her ideas on her intuitive insight, suggested at the turn of the century that "the pineal gland is a distinctive gland of childhood and atrophies later, is there not perhaps some real connection, some indication of hidden truth? Children have a ready belief in God and recognition of him. Christ said 'the Kingdom of Heaven is within you' and except you become as little children you shall not enter into the Kingdom of Heaven."[6]

The tongue is an important organ in psychospiritual integration because it acts like a switch which connects the two currents of "chi"* energy which flow through the body and meet at the base of the spine. The Yang current moves up the spine through the governor, which ends at the top of the mouth. The governor is the main Yang energy channel. Beginning at the tongue and running down the front of the body past the sexual organs to the base of the spine is the main Yin energy channel which is called the conceptual. When the tongue is touching the top of the mouth, the channels are connected and there is a continuous circular flow of energy through the channels which creates a harmonious balance between Yin and Yang energy.

The head corresponds to the Holy of Holies. By moving beyond the throat to the region of the head, the student begins to activate those centers of awareness and wholeness. By harmonizing the flow of Yin and Yang energy, a person creates balance in his energy system. Once the blockages which had prevented energy from flowing past the throat into the head are released, energy can flow into and through the highest energy centers, the sixth and seventh

---

* Chi: otherwise known as Ki, is a Chinese term which refers to the energy that flows through the meridians and chakras. It is often used interchangeably with the term Prana.

chakra whose physical externalization are the pineal and pituitary glands. Once energy can flow without restriction from the base of the spine to the crown of the head, nothing stands in the way of union with the universal field. All barriers have been removed and the student enters the Holy of Holies by having the I AM merge into the ALL, the universal field of energy and consciousness.

Connecting the three sections of the human body is the spine. From the esoteric point of view it is extremely important. In the Taoist tradition it is the route followed by the "Governor." At the base of the spine where the Taoist tells us the two streams of Chi energy enter the human body, the Tantra Sutras tell us the Kundalini Shakti, the coiled serpent energy, is located. In Tantra we are told that this "coiled feminine energy" is the body's most powerful current of psychic energy. As the serpent power is uncoiled, it releases powerful streams of Prana which activate the chakras also located along the spine. The ancient Egyptians believed that the spinal column linked the upper and lower heavens. This metaphor aptly describes the regenerative quality of Kundalini which regenerates a person's consciousness as it uncoils and moves up the spine.

The physical body is rich in esoteric symbolism. The symbols are meant to bring a student into a deeper appreciation of his physical body. In psychospiritual integration the physical body is considered to be the outward expression of the person's subtle bodies.

The symbols draw parallels between the physical body and the subtle bodies, and point to the importance of their harmonious interaction. Indeed, the relationship a person has with the physical world is dependent on their relationship to their physical body. The relationship a person has to their physical body must be honest and nourishing, and the interaction between the physical body and the subtle bodies must not be restricted or blocked. When energy radiates freely between all bodies and when a person is "in their body," when they are fully conscious of their physical body, they will be well on their way to achieving balance, wholeness and unconditional joy.

CHAPTER XI

YOU AND YOUR SUBTLE BODIES

What is essential is invisible to the eye.
—A. de St. Exupery

The Invisible World
When we move from the visible world to the invisible world, we come across many and often conflicting notions of the subtle anatomy of humans. I have compiled my version of the human's subtle anatomy by studying my own subtle bodies and subtle energy system as well as my students,' and by applying techniques I have developed over the years in an attempt to influence them. Where I have been successful, I know that my view was correct. I have also done my best to accommodate my model with those of the major psychological and esoteric systems.

I have found major areas of agreement especially with the Tantric, Yogic, esoteric Taoist and Jungian Systems. These systems largely agree on the subtle anatomy of humans. They see the various subtle bodies as well as the physical body of humans as subfields in the concentration of energy called self . . . each vibrating in a different range of frequencies.

The universal field is divided into four levels or dimensions, each interpenetrating the other and each vibrating

117

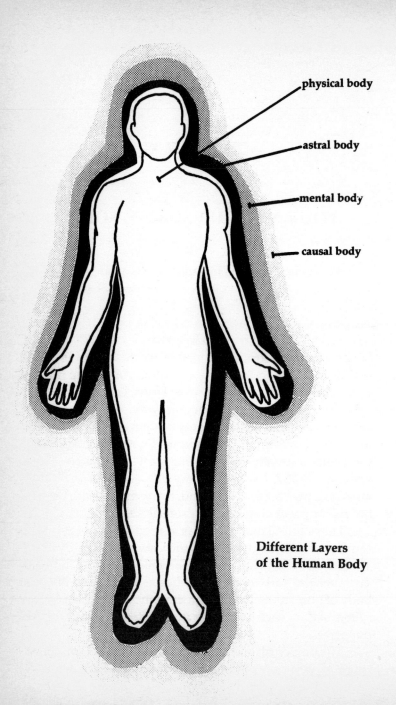

physical body

astral body

mental body

causal body

**Different Layers
of the Human Body**

within a specific range of frequencies. Occupying the lowest level is the physical plane, and the physical body dwells on it. The physical body's point of contact with the subtle bodies which interpenetrate it is the etheric double. It is the vehicle of consciousness for the physical body.

Physical sensations are transmitted to the etheric double from the nervous system by Prana. It is the Prana running along the nerves of the body which generate the sensations. When it comes to emotions, we are dealing with clearly defined ranges of frequencies of Prana. Emotions do not originate in the physical body although they do produce chemical reactions within it. They originate in the astral body (the body of emotions) and are transmitted via the chakras through the etheric double to the physical body.

Each chakra* transmits Prana in a specific range of frequencies. In the same way that specific frequencies of light are interpreted by our brain as different colors, specific frequencies of Prana are interpreted as different emotions or feelings. Each chakra is associated with particular aspects of human awareness. The chakras also act as sensors. They register ranges of frequencies when they encounter them in the outer environment. We sense the emotions of others through the chakras which are situated on the surface of the etheric double, and through the etheric aura which surrounds it.

The Astral Body

The astral body is composed of matter found on the astral plane. Astral matter vibrates at a higher frequency than either physical matter or etheric matter. The astral body connects the mental body to the physical body through its connection to the etheric double.

---

* There are seven chakras which open on the surface of the etheric double. In one of their functions they serve as doorways through which Prana must pass between the astral body and physical body.

It is when the functions of the astral body are integrated and fully conscious that a person can sense energy fields and can function actively through the second attention. In the same way that etheric matter interpenetrates physical matter, and the etheric double interpenetrates the physical body, astral matter interpenetrates etheric matter and the astral body interpenetrates the etheric double and takes on the same size and shape of the etheric double. An important function of the astral body is to provide the physical body (through the etheric double) the energy it needs to remain sentient and to keep it connected to the universal field. It is through the astral body that sensations received via the physical senses are transmitted to the mental body. Every person possesses an astral body although few are aware of it. During times of deep relaxation or meditation, many people have a sense of moving up or down or from side to side which is caused by the astral body being momentarily freed from the rigid confines of the physical body.

The astral body, unlike the etheric double, lies entirely within unconsciousness. Becoming conscious of the astral body, integrating it with the visible parts of self (physical body and etheric double), and controlling its functions is an essential part of the work of psychospiritual integration. When the astral body is fully integrated and its functions become conscious, then a person finds himself with many powers which other people don't seem to possess and which gives him an ability to influence and experience the world in a way that appears almost magical to other people.

The more refined a person is, particularly in the realm of emotions, feelings and preferences, the more refined the astral body will be. When viewed by a clairvoyant, the more refined astral body will have a defined outline (in the same shape as the physical body), its texture will be smooth throughout, and its colors will be bright and clear. The less developed and refined the person is, the more loosely organized and less defined his astral body is. To the clairvoyant, a less refined astral body will appear to be a cloudy mass of astral matter moving chaotically in different directions. It will look dark, coarse and will obscure the outline of the physical body.

The more intense a person feels and the more a person expresses the higher feelings of love, empathy and compassion, the higher will be the vibration of the astral body and the brighter will be its colors. The astral body is the body of emotions, and emotional energy cannot be underestimated in the work of psychospiritual integration. Because of this, it is essential for the student to bring the functions of the astral body under conscious control.

Mutual Attraction

Emotional interaction between people through the medium of astral energy in the form of rays and fields is subject to the principle of mutual attraction. This principle states that like attract like, and a particular emotion or frequency of energy which radiates from a person's astral body attracts the same frequency of energy whether he likes it or not. This law of magnetism or mutual attraction applies to the physical conscious world as well as the subtle worlds of higher vibration. It follows then that although a person might send a particular message consciously such as "I want to be a success," this message can be nullified because on the astral level he might be forever subverting himself by sending a contrary message, by projecting a contrary range of energy.

A person's unconscious reservoirs of fear, anger and pain are stored in the astral body and the etheric aura which surrounds it. They vibrate and flow from there into the environment, and this unconscious and largely uncontrolled flow of energy brings a person comparable energy in return. Their fear attracts fear, their pain attracts pain, and their anger attracts anger. So, although a person might seek success, joy or love consciously, unconsciously anger, pain, resentment, jealousy, or the fear of success, etc., might effectively prevent him from achieving his conscious desire.

It is through the astral body that a person senses the mood or feelings of another person or the climate of a room or physical environment. This ability is developed to one degree or another in everyone, and its cultivation is very important for us. It is through our ability to feel our impact on the environment and the environment's impact on us that we can know our rightful position in the world on a moment to moment basis.

Whether other frequencies of energy encountered in the world are sympathetic with our own energy or discordant, it is important for us to be aware of what frequencies of energy enter our personal energy field because much of the harmony and disharmony in our lives can be accounted for by living in an atmosphere of either harmonious or discordant human energy fields.

If the people you surround yourself with have reservoirs of feelings, in particular pain, anger, and fear repressed and stored within their astral body, then you can be adversely affected by these fields, because energy is released from them through the astral body and this energy will be picked up by your astral body. No amount of conscious suppression is sufficient to block these unconscious emissions completely. If a person doesn't release his/her repressed feelings consciously, they will remain within the storage areas of the astral body. Notwithstanding his/her best intentions, these feelings will affect people around him/her and dispose people who can't process them against him/her.

One of the biggest problems people have in understanding energy fields is the issue of whether energy in the form of thoughts and emotions come spontaneously from their own energy fields or whether they are coming from another field and are entering their energy field either through conscious or unconscious projection. Below are some guidelines which will help you to determine what feelings and thoughts (frequencies of Prana) are generated from your personal energy field and which enter your field from outside.

1. Thought precedes emotion: If you begin to feel something not related to what you are thinking about, it is probably not your feeling, and the feeling is coming from an outside energy field.

2. Thoughts and feelings out of the context of what you are doing at the moment generally are not your own.

3. Heavy feelings that press on you from the outside are not your feelings. They are being projected to you from an outside field.

4. Feelings and thoughts that hammer at you—even when you want to get rid of them, are not your own; they come from outside your field.

5. Sudden and dramatic emotional changes are caused by entering discordant energy fields.

6. Changes, accusations, badgering and the perpetual charge, "You are wrong," don't originate in your personal energy field.

7. Sudden weakness or exhaustion as well as confusion or anxiety come from discordant energy fields.

8. Physical experiences, heat, pressures, thrills, etc.,

which are out of context to what you are doing are generated by outside fields.

The Mental Body

The astral body is interpenetrated by the mental body. The mental body gives and receives information, and gets its nourishment from the mental plane. It is composed of finer matter than that found on the astral plane. It is from the transmutation of spiritual matter (transmutation takes place when spiritual matter has its frequency vibration lowered) that the mental body is formed. The mental body connects the astral body with the causal body (spiritual body), the body of highest vibration.

The mental body deals with what in Sanskrit is called *Rupa* or thought forms. It deals with concrete thoughts, as well as intuition, and the various paranormal abilities such as clairvoyance and clairaudience. The mental body does this by processing abstract thought which originates in the spiritual body and applying it to concrete situations.

The process can be linked to the formation and disintegration of bubbles which originate deep within a body of water; the body of water represents the unconscious, the almost hidden nature of the I AM. The invisible contents of the bubbles come from an even deeper and unknowable source from within the universal field. As long as the bubbles remain under water, they are within the unconscious mind and remain largely inaccessible. But when the bubbles reach the surface, they cross over an invisible threshold between the unconscious mind and the conscious mind. At the critical moment they burst. If at that moment the person is truly aware and has integrated and balanced intuitive thought with rational thought, he can access the information and instead of it being lost, it is captured by the conscious mind where it is immediately applied to practical, concrete situations. If conscious mental activity is not inte-

grated with unconscious mental activity, then this transmutation of abstract thought into more concrete thought is
impossible, because there is a gulf between the unconscious,
intuitive and the rational, conscious mind.

Because of its intimate relationship with the astral
body, the mental body's true function can become distorted
when it is influenced by sentimentality which originates in
the astral body. (Sentimentality is caused by an over-
abundance of astral energy.) If this occurs, the mental body
becomes dominated by thoughts which are associated with
physical well-being and comfort. As a result, the mental
body will have its normal function disrupted. When this
happens, the mental body becomes grounded in mundane
affairs. Its main function then becomes rational problem
solving based on the survival principle that the greatest
good is what ensures physical survival and personal well-
being. However, this is a distortion of the true nature of the
mental body whose main purpose is to be the mental vehicle for the I AM.

The mental body can be influenced in three ways: It
can be influenced from above, when abstract thought enters
the mental body from the causal body. This sets in motion
the matter of the mental body and this in turn transmutes
the abstraction into something comprehensible, that being
concrete thought. This form of thought is intuitive in nature
and normally comes as insight or intuition. Thoughts of this
type are usually experienced as pictures or sounds. In its
highest form, thoughts of this type often produce what the
Greeks called *catharsis*, a sudden and dramatic insight into
the truth of something. Catharsis is normally thought of as a
rare glimpse into the true nature of things. However, I have
found that catharsis can be cultivated and can become a
common and even programmable experience which can be
used for creative problem solving.

The second way the mental body can be influenced is

by the physical body and astral body. If we work from the physical plane, the process follows this rough outline. First, the physical body is stimulated by something from the physical environment. From the physical body and the senses, the sensation or information is carried to the etheric double which is influenced and begins to vibrate. The subtle matter of the etheric body influences the astral body which registers the sensation, and the sensation is relayed via Prana to the mental body which reacts to it by vibrating. This vibration stimulates the creation of thought. Thoughts which move in this direction can end in the mental body. If they do, they take on the form of verbal thought. When this process is continual, what is created is the internal dialogue. If there is an even modest degree of integration between the causal body and the mental body, then the vibration will pass through the mental body, touch the causal body and create a ripple in it which rebounds and heightens the vibration of the original thought. When this is the case, the vibration will return to the mental body, not in the form of verbal thought, but in the form of visual or musical thought.

The third way that the mental body is influenced is by thoughts which come directly from the minds of other people. Once a person has learned to still even a portion of the internal dialogue, he/she will begin to realize that many of the thoughts that appear to come spontaneously from his own mind actually are projected from the minds of others. By paying attention to the quality of his thoughts, a person can learn to discriminate and distinguish which thoughts are his own, and which are not.

A person who has developed discrimination can even discern the origin and quality of thought entering his mind. He can then choose to reject thoughts which are harmful to himself and accept thoughts which are beneficial. After a while, if the mental body is working in its full capacity, it will attract only beneficial, energizing thoughts and will automatically reject those thoughts which are enervating or otherwise harmful.

Detachment

Much of people's difficulties begin in the mental body, because the mental body is usually far less integrated than the functions of the lower bodies. The average person normally identifies with his physical body, its feelings and ego-centered consciousness. The integrated person, however, has retrieved the full capabilities of the mental body and can assert enormous power in the realm of concentration and will. He can even separate mental functions from the functions of the astral and physical body. By doing this, he achieves detachment which is of enormous importance in our work. Detachment should not be confused with fragmentation which is the result of separation. Detachment is achieved when an integrated person experiences himself as the union of selves. As long as a person identifies with the lower bodies (the astral, etheric and physical bodies) he cannot achieve detachment. When a person achieves detachment, he experiences a far greater personal freedom and flexibility, because fears and desires, which are functions of his lower bodies, have little or no effect on him and his behavior, and decisions are based only on his intuition and a clear perception of their Dharma.

The Causal Body

The spiritual or immortal part of man, the part which persists throughout man's entire evolution, goes by many names. The ancient Egyptians named it *Za*. In the Upanishad, it is called the *Atman* and in Tantra it is called *Karana sarira*. The Theosophists took the idea of Karana Sarira and called the divine part of man the causal body. When dealing with the causal body, we move beyond the realm of personality to a divine essence which is imperishable and indescribable. Ramakrishna, when asked, "How does the Lord dwell in the body?" answered, "He dwells in the body like the plug of a syringe—that is, in the body, and yet apart from it."[1] It is important for us to remember that the causal body, unlike the other subtle bodies, is part of us and yet not part of us; it is, as it were, the divine thread which keeps us connected to the All and which imbues us with its essence.

The law of interpenetration explains the location of our causal body as well as the bodies of lower vibrations in relation to each other.

The higher bodies fit into the lower bodies like a hand fits into a glove. When we come to the causal body, however, we have a somewhat different situation. The causal body not only fits into the mental body, it is interpenetrated directly by the universal field. Through the causal body, a person participates in the universal field and is united to everything else in the universe. On the causal level, there is no possibility that union can be disrupted. Fragmentation begins on the level of mind in the mental body and it is transmuted downwards. The causal body cannot under any circumstance become separated from the universal field of energy and consciousness. The causal or spiritual body is the divine spark within us; it is the body of highest vibration.

It rests in the universal field and receives its nourishment directly from the universal field. It has never and can never become separated from the universal field. From the spiritual plane the most radiant and profound spiritual energy enters a human being. From there the energy is transmuted by having its frequency lowered for use on the lower planes by the lower bodies: the mental body, the astral body, the etheric body and the physical body.

Accepting our union with the universal field, the existence of the causal body is essential for the work of psychospiritual integration. Because union is the primordial state of the universe, it exists even today and will continue to exist for eternity. Everything that is, is a manifestation of the All and as a result is part of the All. For us to believe that we have a separate existence outside of the All or that we can be whole independent of the All is as silly as the finger thinking it can exist apart from the hand, or that it can be defined outside the context of the whole body.

> The universe consisting of both the decaying
> and undecaying states,
> the manifested and the unmanifested forms,
> the effect and the cause,
> is held by the Lord of the universe (God)
> It is He Himself,
> who for enjoying His own creation,
> imprisons himself in every being.
> He again after knowing his own true self,
> frees himself from all fetters
> (of this mortal world).[2]

CHAPTER XII

THE CHAKRAS AND CHAKRA MEDITATIONS

The unknown is the superfluous part of the average man, and it is superfluous because the average man doesn't have enough energy to grasp it.
—Carlos Castaneda
The Fire From Within

The subtle energy system is composed of the nadis which conduct Prana through the subtle bodies, the three auras (the reservoirs of energy surrounding the four bodies), the Hara, located three fingers below the navel (the fulcrum from which everything else is balanced), and the seven chakras.

The seven chakras are energy centers, gates and transformers, located along the spine and up into the head which connect the nadis with the three auras surrounding the physical and subtle bodies. Like antennas, they pick up or sense the complete range of energy entering a person's personal energy field. The personal energy field extends outwards in layers; at its greatest extent it averages about 26 feet in all directions beyond the surface of the physical body.

The chakras process and distribute energy entering them through the different nadis and auras. What's more, they transform the frequencies into different sensations, comprehensible to a human being, namely thought, emotion and physical sensation. The chakras do this in the same way that the eye refracts light. When different frequencies of light which enter the brain are interpreted by the brain as different colors, the chakras, by refracting subtle energy, in effect break it down into particular impressions that make an impact on a person. Moreover, each chakra serves as a channel for a range of frequencies of energy entering a person's personal energy field.

Beyond this, the chakras act as transformers, organs of transmutation. The subtle energy system can be likened to an electrical circuit. Energy enters the subtle energy system from different energy sources where it is stepped up or down by the chakras. By having its frequency transmuted in this way, the energy can perform whatever functions are necessary on a particular level of causation. Transmutation can occur when any body is in an energy deficit position. When energy is needed by either the physical body or one of the subtle bodies, it will be transferred from the adjacent body by having its frequency transmuted by the appropriate chakra. This is precisely what happens in spiritual healing when excess energy from the astral and mental bodies is transmuted for use by the physical body to heal itself.

Transmutation is not limited to one direction. It can occur in the four directions in which energy flows through the subtle energy system: up, down, in and out. Energy is transmuted by the chakras as it moves down from the seventh chakra which is the gate through which the highest frequencies enter a person from the causal plane. Energy from the physical body can be transmuted for use in the higher bodies; energy from surrounding energy fields can be transmuted as it passes through a person's auras and enters the particular chakra which is sensitive to its frequency. Finally, a person can project rays of energy from his/her chakras and with these rays can transmute energy in another person's energy system by stepping it up or down.

Hiroshi Motoyama tells us "thus the chakra is seen to be an intermediary for energy transfer and conversion between two neighbouring dimensions of being, as well as a center facilitating the energy conversion between a body and its corresponding mind."[1]

According to most authorities, the subtle bodies of man contain seven chakras and they open (or we can say their lotus appear) on the surface of the etheric double. By their nature, the chakras are inter-dimensional, because they are energy converters. Each chakra straddles at least two levels of causation, the physical/astral, astral/mental, and mental/causal. We must remember, however, that the division of the universe into planes is a simplification to facilitate our understanding of a multi-dimensional universe.

Of the seven energy centers, two originate in the head and five at the spinal column. The energy centers must all be open and in balance if a person is to experience wholeness and unconditional joy. Unfortunately, few people have their chakras open and in balance. Instead, for the vast majority, the chakras vary in activity depending on how conscious a person has become on each plane of causation at any given time, and how blocked each chakra is because of stress or fear. These conditions vary widely within the life of each individual, depending on their level of integration in a given situation.

An easy way to determine which chakras are blocked is to simply pay attention to which parts of your body get tight, or begin to hurt when you are overloaded and can't process all the energy flowing through your subtle energy system. If, for example, you get a headache when you are overloaded, it is your sixth chakra, the third eye, which is blocked. If you develop a tightness in your throat, discover a "frog" in your throat, or the back of your neck or shoulders get tight and begin to hurt, you have a blockage at the fifth chakra, the throat chakra. If your heart begins to pound or you get palpitations in your heart center when you are stressed, then the blockage is in the fourth chakra, the heart center.

When you feel tightness in your stomach or your stomach begins to ache, the restriction is in the third chakra, the solar plexus center. Blockages in the second chakra, the sexual center, can manifest as either an ache in the intestines, problems with digestion, problems in the urinary tract or sexual dysfunction. For women there can be a disruption in menstruation when the second chakra is blocked. A blockage in the first chakra at the base of the spine can also manifest as digestive problems or difficulties with the bowel movement.

There is a relationship between the health and activity of specific chakras, a person's behavior and the quality of their relationships. A person whose sixth and seventh chakras are open and functioning normally but whose heart chakra is for some reason blocked will have difficulty expressing strong feelings and will concentrate on the mental life instead of seeking out satisfying relationships. A person whose solar plexus is blocked might be balanced everywhere else in life. He/she may be able to love and to engage in healthy fulfilling sex, but the sense of belonging, contentment and ability to make commitments will be blocked and he/she will have difficulty sustaining relationships.

As a general rule, the more evolved a person is, the more active the higher chakras become. It is rare, however, to find a person who is evolved enough to work predominantly through the sixth and seventh chakra while having the lower five open and balanced as well. So it is unusual to find someone who doesn't feel an emptiness deep within themselves. Most people are largely stuck in their animal nature and live predominantly through their first five chakras.

According to Alice Bailey, at the current state of human evolution, "the throat center is beginning to make itself felt with the head and heart centers still asleep."[2]

The Muladhara Chakra

The first chakra is located at the base of the spine in the area of the coccyx. In Sanskrit it is called the *Muladhara* chakra. *Mula* means root, *adhara* support. It glows with a fiery red color. The first chakra is associated with the Earth, with the qualities of resistance and solidity. It opens downward in the direction of the Earth, and this in itself would indicate its importance in connecting a person to their physical environment. Through the first chakra, energy from the Earth enters the subtle energy system and it is through the first chakra that a person feels their connection to the Earth. When the first chakra is functioning normally, a person is aware that their life is not separate from the life of the planet which gave birth to their physical body and where at death it eventually returns.

The first chakra is particularly important in psychospiritual integration because it is the seat of Kundalini, and in Taoist tradition, the starting point for the three principal meridians. We must consider it also as one end of a system that at the opposite end opens at the seventh chakra. To maintain the proper pressure within the system, the first chakra must be opened and balanced with the seventh chakra. Furthermore, each chakra has the responsibility to maintain the health of a particular section of the physical body. The first chakra controls the horizontal section of the body from just below the buttocks to a point just above the sexual organs. It controls excretion and the digestion of food. The health and proper function of the small intestine and colon is dependent on its proper function. It has an influence on sexual well-being, especially in men because of its influence over the prostate gland. Some authorities claim it governs the functioning of the kidneys as well.

Muladhara Meditation

Each chakra controls a certain range of frequencies of energy flowing into and out of if from either the physical or one or more of the subtle bodies. It isn't enough to understand this phenomena intellectually or even to experience it on the unconscious level. It is important to consciously experience and to consciously be able to regulate the energy as it radiates into, through and out of each particular chakra. I've created a series of meditations designed to help you consciously experience, regulate and integrate the functions of the chakras with each other and with the other organs of the subtle energy system. In the Muladhara meditation I want you to feel the energy flowing through the first chakra. Then get in touch with that center of consciousness which is your earth-like nature and become that consciousness to the exclusion of everything else.

To begin the Muladhara meditation, it is first necessary to get in touch with the energy of the Muladhara center and increase it. By increasing the level of energy it will be easier to experience the energy in the chakra, and then the consciousness which is a manifestation of the sub-field created by the chakra. To start, find a comfortable position, preferably with your back straight, close your eyes and begin the Yogic Breath. Breathe deeply through your nose without separation between inhalation and exhalation, and feel yourself relaxing. Take your time and let yourself become conscious of your body. This is easiest to do if you pay attention to your breathing for about five minutes, allowing it to get deeper and more rhythmic with each breath. After about five minutes bring your attention to your first chakra at the base of your spine. It's all right if you don't know exactly where it is. Bring your attention to where you think it is. Then begin breathing in and out from your first chakra.

I want you to feel that on every inhalation the breath does not stop at the bottom of your lungs but that it continues flowing down all the way to the base of your spine. Without separation between inhalation and exhalation, breathe out naturally through your nose. On each exhalation feel as if the energy at the base of your spine is growing stronger. You will feel the energy as a heat and intensity which will become more powerful on each exhalation. As it grows stronger, visualize the energy there as a ball of fiery, red energy. Continue both experiencing and visualizing the energy growing brighter for two or three minutes. Let your consciousness, which for most people is centered somewhere around the shoulders and neck, move downward until it reaches the base of your spine and becomes centered in the ball of energy. Become the ball of energy and feel yourself being drawn downward into the Earth.

As this happens, pay attention to how you feel physically, emotionally and mentally. For some of you there will be profound changes on each level. Some of you will experience imagery associated with the Earth, imagery associated with the cycles of life, death and rebirth. Some students report experiencing feelings of continuity and rapport with other life forms or feelings of security, partnership and belonging associated with Nature and Mother Earth.

By doing this exercise repeatedly, you will learn about different aspects of your earth-like nature and your connection and interdependent relationship with the Earth. I would suggest that you take at least 10 minutes for this part of the meditation. After 10 minutes or when you are satisfied, take a deep breath through your nose, and as you exhale mentally repeat, "Every time I come to this level of consciousness I learn to use more of my mind more creatively." Next let your breathing return to normal, release the ball of energy at the base of your spine and the imagery associated with the first chakra. Then mentally return to the room and relax. After a few moments, begin to count mentally from one to five and when you reach the number five, open your eyes. You will feel wide awake, perfectly relaxed and better than you did before.

The Svadhisthana Chakra

The second chakra is called *Svadhisthana*. *Sva* means "that which is its self; which belongs to itself" and *Dhisthana* means "its actual place." The importance of this definition for our work is the recognition that it is primarily through the second chakra that a person experiences the deep feelings associated with their physical manifestation. The chakra is situated just above the genitals. It regulates sexual energy, which is far more than mere physical sexuality or eroticism. It is the seat of creativity through which a person experiences the childlike wonder and excitement of the manifest universe. It is from the second chakra that a person experiences the world as a magical place. It is also where a man experiences his intrinisic masculinity and a woman her intrinsic femininity. It is rare for a child to restrict the flow of energy through their second chakra, and that is why until they reach puberty children retain their childlike innocence. But with all the taboos, and restrictions relating to sexuality, the proper flow of energy through this vital center is rarely seen in adults.

Innocence and wonder are not lost because of sexual maturation as is commonly thought. On the contrary, they are lost because of blockages in the second chakra which begin for most people during puberty.

In the course of working with people I have often heard statements by my students such as: "I want to be an integrated person" or, "I want to become a whole, self-realized being." But I have found that ultimately there are no self-realized people. There are only self-realized men and self-realized women.

Remembrance, recollection and reunion cannot be achieved until a person regains the sense of being a man or a woman. This can only be achieved when a person reclaims that most human part of him/herself: the second chakra and the subfield associated with it.

According to yogic texts, the Svadhisthana chakra is located just above and in front of the first chakra, the Muladhara. It controls many of the pelvic organs including the urinary tract and sexual organs. It also influences the other organs of digestion and excretion, but because of its proximity to the first chakra, it is difficult to separate its functions in relation to the physical body from those of the Muladhara. In Tantra, we are told that the Svadhisthana governs the flow of Prana through the five vertebrae of the sacrum. Tantric texts also suggest that the Svadhisthana chakra governs the principle of taste and it is associated with the element water.

Because of its proximity to the Hara, the second chakra plays a vital function in the proper flow and distribution of Prana.

In the Svadhisthana meditation, try to get in touch with that center of consciousness which embodies your magical, sensual nature, that nature which is full of wonder and excitement, which sees life in everything else and participates in the ongoing ecstasy of creation. Become conscious of that part of your nature to the exclusion of everything else.

Svadhisthana Meditation

To begin the Svadhisthana meditation, find a comfortable position with your back straight. Close your eyes and begin breathing yogically. Breathe deeply through your nose without separation between inhalation and exhalation and feel yourself relaxing. Take your time and become conscious of your body by following your breath for about five minutes. After about five minutes, bring your attention to your second chakra, right above your sexual organs. Then bring your breath to your second chakra. On each inhalation, feel the energy centered in your sexual organs increasing. You will feel it as a heat and intensity which will grow stronger on each inhalation. As it grows stronger, visualize the energy there as a ball of orange energy. Experience and visualize it growing stronger and brighter for about two or three minutes.

Next, feel your consciousness move downward until it reaches a point just above your sexual organs and feel your consciousness centered in that ball of energy. Become the ball of energy and feel yourself begin to radiate outward from that center through your body and then into the outer environment. Feel the magic and the sense of wonder which is a manifestation of the energy which radiates from the second chakra. Pay attention to how you feel physically, emotionally and mentally. Some of you may feel spontaneous bursts of energy running up and down your spine or through your body. These are called *Kriyas* in Sanskrit. They are normal; enjoy them. You might feel them as a warm current of energy, or vibrations flowing through your body. These sensations are associated with an increased energy flow. Pay attention to the changes you experience—observe them, but don't try to influence them. After a short time you will begin to experience imagery associated with the second chakra. Some of it might be sexual at first but if you don't identify with it or get attached to it, the sexual imagery will pass and it will be replaced with pictures associated with the creative process.

Take at least 10 minutes for this part of the meditation. After about 10 minutes or when you are satisfied, take a deep breath through your nose and as you exhale mentally repeat, "Every time I come to this level of consciousness I learn to use more of my mind in more creative ways." Then let your breathing return to normal, release the ball of energy by your second chakra and the imagery associated with it and mentally return to the room and relax.

After a few moments, begin to count mentally from one to five and when you reach the number five, open your eyes. You will feel wide awake, perfectly relaxed and better than you did before.

The Manipura Chakra

The third chakra is called *Manipura* which in Sanskrit means "city of jewels." It is located by the solar plexus and is the seat of personality. It is responsible for the assimilation of food, and it controls the horizontal section of the physical body from a point about two fingers above the solar plexus downward to a point about two fingers above the navel. We are told that when the chakra is open and functioning normally a person obtains calmness ... and is even able to retain calmness in times of distress.

The third chakra has control over the solar plexus ganglia which plays an important part in a person's relationship to the world, to people, places and things. Our ability to connect, to belong, to make long-term intimate associations, the love of home, family, country, etc. are all associated with the energy of the third chakra. What's more, the feelings of contentment and trust are also regulated by the solar plexus. The extraordinary difference between the solar plexus chakra and the other chakras (in particular the heart chakra which controls the four strong emotions), is its consistency. The energy radiating from it is the most consistent and uniform in frequency in the subtle energy system. As the diagram below illustrates, the frequencies which radiate through the heart vary greatly in amplitude. If represented graphically, they would resemble the diagram below:

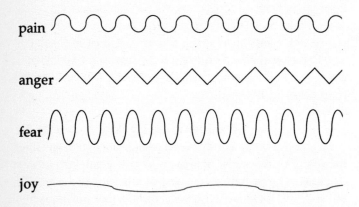

The frequencies associated with the solar plexus are far more consistent. There is a reliability and predictability about them. The frequencies radiating from the solar plexus would more accurately resemble the graph below:

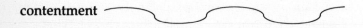

In regard to long-term intimate relationships, it has been my experience that the love that comes through the heart is not sufficiently consistent to forge a bond complete enough and strong enough for both partners to sustain the relationship indefinitely. For a relationship to last and for it to grow in trust, both parties must connect from the solar plexus center as well as from the heart center. The energy from the solar plexus is the energy which supports commitment and trust, and these two radiations of energy must flow freely if people hope to stay together for a lifetime.

By disrupting the proper function of the third chakra, a person inadvertantly prevents energy from moving past the diaphragm. As a result it cannot be transmuted from more mundane frequencies to those associated with the subtle bodies and spiritual awareness. The unfortunate result is that by blocking the free radiation of energy from the solar plexus, a person cuts her/himself off from the conscious awareness of the subtle bodies and the I AM radiating from the center of his/her being. As a result, proper ego development is disrupted and ego develops exclusively in consciousness. Fear of the unloved others and fear of reliving the pain of separation experienced in childhood are the primary cause of blockages in the third chakra. That is why reservoirs of fear are most often located in the abdomen.

The Manipura Meditation

In the Manipura meditation, you have the opportunity to get in touch with the awareness which transcends conscious mind. In this meditation you will get in touch with that transcendental self which allows you to participate and empathize with other people, and to connect deeply with them. By experiencing the radiations of the third chakra consciously, you will transcend "me" concerns and experience the selflessness which permits you to connect with other people and to feel the deep contentment associated with that connection.

To begin the Manipura meditation, find a comfortable position with your back straight, close your eyes and begin the Yogic breath by breathing deeply through your nose without separation between inhalation and exhalation. As you breathe yogically, feel yourself relaxing. Become conscious of your body by paying attention to your breath for about five minutes. After about five minutes, bring your mental attention to your third chakra located just below the breastbone and begin breathing in and out from it. On each inhalation you will feel the energy in the solar plexus growing stronger. You will feel it as a heat and intensity. As the energy grows stronger, visualize it as a ball of golden yellow energy. Visualize and experience it growing brighter for two or three minutes. Next, feel your consciousness move downward until it becomes centered in the ball of energy. Become the ball of energy and feel yourself radiating outward from it, first through your body and then into the outer environment. As you radiate, you will feel yourself beginning to melt.

You will feel yourself becoming watery and fluid. As your consciousness radiates from that center, you will feel a profound empathy. This empathy, which is the product of trust and contentment, will permit you to feel compassion for the pain and suffering of others as well as for yourself. Surrender to these feelings and let them flow through you. Take about 10 minutes for this part of the meditation. After about 10 minutes or when you feel satisfied, take a deep breath through your nose and as you exhale mentally repeat, "Every time I come to this level of consciousness I learn to use more of my mind in more creative ways." Then let your breathing return to normal, release the ball of energy from your third chakra and the imagery associated with it, and mentally return to the room and relax. After a few moments, count mentally from one to five and when you reach the number five, open your eyes. You will feel wide awake, perfectly relaxed and better than you did before.

The Anahata Chakra
The fourth chakra is called *Anahata* which in Sanskrit means "unbeater." It is located at the eighth cervical ver-

tebra of the spine opposite the region of the heart. The chakra is associated with the element air and with touch. It controls the horizontal area of the physical body extending from the collar bones to a point about two fingers above the solar plexus. Crossing over from Manipura to Anahata is a difficult one.

By moving beyond the diaphragm, a person moves from the outer courtyard to the inner courtyard of the body temple. By taking this step, a person begins to recognize that "self" is beyond definition ... that it is constantly changing as it adapts to a constantly shifting spectrum of possibilities. Which self is predominant at any particular time is determined by the person's energy level and the circumstances created by the inner and outer environments to which the person must adjust.

The heart chakra is associated with compassion and healing, and in this capacity it radiates a bright emerald green color. In its transcendental aspect, the heart chakra is the source of light and love; not only of human love, but agape love, the Divine love which the New Testament so poetically describes as "rivers of living water."

Leadbeater tells us that the heart chakra, when awakened, endows a person with the power to "sympathize with the vibrations of other astral entities so that he could instinctively understand something of their feeling."[3] This is simply another way of saying that by opening the heart center, a person achieves the ability to sense energy fields and atmospheres. Moreover, by opening the heart chakra, a person can affect the fields of other people in a positive way by projecting energy to them through the Anahata Center. This is essentially what chakra healing is. Through the combined effort of the heart center and Ajna center (third eye), a person can project rays of energy to another person and this energy will have a healing effect on them. The thymus gland is located just over the heart chakra. It has a regulatory effect on the physical bodies' immunological system, and if the normal function of the heart chakra is blocked so will be the function of the thymus gland. As a consequence, the immunological system will be suppressed.

The heart chakra is the gateway to the astral body, and in this role it can be thought of as the regulator of a person's emotional life. The heart chakra regulates the quality and interactions of joy, pain, fear and anger. However, for these emotions to flow properly and to be released normally the chakra must be open and in balance with the other chakras. If it is blocked in any way, then emotions will be distorted. If a person blocks the flow of a so-called negative emotion because of fear, in effect they block the normal flow of all emotions, including joy which, when it radiates outwardly, becomes love. Moreover, when the heart chakra is blocked, a person finds it difficult to stay balanced because energy cannot flow properly between the physical and subtle bodies. As a result, a person loses touch with the physical body because the sensations coming from the astral body through the etheric double don't have access to the physical body. The numbness of the physical body is the physical externalization of numbness in a person's emotional body and emotional life.

In classical Yogic texts the heart chakra is described as the gateway to the soul. Centuries ago, the Yogis recognized that the All through the agency of the I AM has access to the subtle and physical bodies of man through the heart chakra.

"Herein is love not that we loved God but that he loved us . . . God is love and he that dwelleth in love dwelleth in God and god in him."[4]

It is through the heart chakra that the All has access to a person in his/her multiplicity. Brother Lawrence describes the experience of awakening the Anahata and allowing himself to be reunited with the All through love.

I have quitted all forms of devotion and set prayers but those to which my state obliges me. And I make it my business only to persevere in his Holy presence where I keep myself by a single attention, and a general fond regard to God, which I may call an actual presence of God, or to speak better, an habitual silent and secret conversation with God, which often causes me joy and raptures, inwardly and sometimes also outwardly so great that I am forced to use means to moderate them and prevent their appearance to others.[5]

Anahata Meditation

In the Anahata meditation you will get in touch with that manifestation of self which is a function of the heart chakra. To begin this meditation, find a comfortable position with your back straight. Close your eyes and begin breathing yogically. Breathe deeply through your nose without separation between inhalation and exhalation, and feel yourself relaxing. Take your time and become conscious of your body by following your breath for about five minutes. After five minutes, bring your attention to your fourth chakra at the center of your breastbone. Then bring your breath to your fourth chakra. On each inhalation feel the energy centered in your heart chakra grow stronger. You will feel it as a heat and intensity which will grow more powerful on each inhalation. As it grows stronger, visualize the energy there as a ball of emerald green light. Experience and visualize it growing stronger and brighter for about two or three minutes. Feel your consciousness move downward until it reaches a point at the center of your chest and feel your consciousness centered in the ball of energy. Then become the ball of energy and feel yourself radiate outward from that center through your body and then into the outer environment.

Feel the transcendent love which radiates through the heart chakra and pay attention to how you feel physically, emotionally and mentally. The more you are centered in the heart, the more you will feel the "mystic heart" of Christ in you. As the rivers of living water radiate through your heart, your whole body will pulsate and searing currents of energy will shoot everywhere: down your legs until they cause the soles of your feet to vibrate, through your arms and hands, and up to the top of your head.

You will experience a warmth that pulsates rhythmically from your heart and fills your whole body. As you surrender to the energy radiating through your heart, you will experience compassion and unconditional love for yourself as well as everyone else, and you will experience the condition which Jesus described as the peace that passes all understanding.

Take at least ten minutes for this part of the meditation. After about ten minutes or when you are satisfied, take a deep breath through your nose and as you exhale mentally repeat, "Every time I come to this level of consciousness I learn to use more of my mind in more creative ways." Then let your breath return to normal, release the ball of energy by your fifth chakra and any imagery associated with it and mentally return to the room and relax. After a few moments, count from one to five and when you reach the number five, open your eyes. You will feel wide awake, perfectly relaxed and better than you did before.

The Visuddha Chakra

The fifth chakra is called *Visuddha* which means "pure" in Sanskrit. It extends from the base of the neck by the third cervical vertebra, just below the medula oblongata to a point in the throat by the Adam's apple. It is associated with the element *Akasa* (which relates to things ethereal) as well as with hearing and the principle of the sound. It controls the horizontal region of the physical body from the midpoint of the nose to the collar bones. Once it is activated, a person becomes conscious of their mental body. We are told in some Yogic texts that it represents the intellectual body or *vijnanamaya kosa*. By this the yogis mean that once the throat chakra is activated, a person is able to separate the functions of the mental body from those of the lower bodies, astral, etheric and physical. By doing this, a person achieves detachment. The power of understanding increases. Clarity is achieved along with a clear perception of Dharma. Alice Bailey tells us: "These centers vary in activity according to the evolutionary status of the individual. In some people certain centers may be relatively quiescent . . . In average humanity the throat center is beginning to make itself felt with the head and heart centers still asleep."[6] The throat chakra is associated with the color blue. Leadbeater suggests that "its general effect is silvery and gleaming . . . as of moonlight upon rippling water."[7]

By activating the fifth chakra, a person becomes aware for the first time that the internal worlds are real worlds, and that as human beings we exist on the subtle worlds and physical world simultaneously. The throat chakra controls a person's ability to express him/herself fully and creatively. It transmits the intent of a soul (astral and mental bodies). Yogic texts tell us that it controls *Udana Vayu* which is the form of Prana which permits vocal expression. But Udana Vaya controls more than just speaking. It controls the entire area of the throat, neck and face. And because of this facial expression, gestures and even the amount of personal space a person demands is dependent on Udana Vayu. Thus the chakra is synonymous with personal integrity. Once Prana can flow through the spine past the throat chakra, a person can stand firm in the face of opposition. He/she can say no. It is because of the throat chakra's unique ability to transmute other forms of human energy into unconditional joy that this becomes possible.

The throat chakra can be likened to a watershed. Heavier frequencies of energy, including anger, pain and fear, moving through it from the lower chakras are automatically transmuted into unconditional joy. All forms of energy from the lower four chakras (the quality or quantity of energy does not matter) can be processed and transmuted by the fifth chakra in this way. The energy, after it is transmuted, can be used to nourish the physical and subtle bodies. What's more, any surplus energy will radiate outward filling the environment with joy and surrounding the persons whose throat chakra is open with a charismatic glow.

It is by awakening the throat chakra that a person transcends fear. Once fear is transmuted, the I AM can emerge and a person can express him/herself completely in all situations. It is then that a person fully understands what the Apostle Paul meant when he said: "For God hath not given us the spirit of fear, but of power and of love, and of a sound mind."[8]

Visuddha Meditation

In the Visuddha meditation, you will get in touch with the joy that is a manifestation of the transforming quality of the fifth chakra. To begin the Visuddha meditation, find a comfortable position with your back straight. Close your eyes and begin breathing yogically. Breathe deeply through your nose without separation between inhalation and exhalation, and feel yourself relaxing. Take your time and become conscious of your body by following your breath for about five minutes. After about five minutes, bring your attention to your fifth chakra at your throat. Then bring your breath to your fifth chakra. On each inhalation feel the energy centered in your throat chakra growing stronger.

You will feel it as a heat and intensity. Visualize the energy there as a ball of blue light. Experience and visualize it growing stronger and brighter for about two or three minutes.

Feel your consciousness move downward until it is centered in the ball of energy. Then become the ball of energy and feel yourself radiating outward from that center through your body and into the outer environment. Feel yourself in your fearless character . . . noble and full of courage; experiencing the integrity of choosing yourself at every moment. Feel an inner affirmation coming through you—an affirmation which says "yes" to life at every moment. The more you are centered in your throat, the more triumphant you will feel. Without diminishing anyone else, your life will be victorious at every moment.

If you wish, you can mentally repeat the affirmation, "At last I am free" over and over to yourself. As you experience your victory on all levels of causation simultaneously, you will feel streams of energy shooting up your spine. As they pass your throat chakra, they will become currents of unconditional joy. Accept your victory. By doing so, you will be fulfilling your Dharma by being yourself completely at every moment.

Take at least ten minutes for this part of the meditation. After about ten minutes or when you are satisfied, take a deep breath through your nose and as you exhale mentally repeat, "Every time I come to this level of consciousness, I learn to use more of my mind in more creative ways." Then let your breath return to normal, release the ball of energy by your fifth chakra and any imagery associated with it, and relax. After a few moments, count mentally from one to five and when you reach the number five, open your eyes. You will feel wide awake, perfectly relaxed and better than you did before.

The Ajna Center

The sixth chakra is called *Ajna* which in Sanskrit means "command." It is sometimes called Shiva Netra which means Shiva's eye or *Jnana* Netra—the eye of wisdom. Some classical texts identify it with the pituitary gland. It is located between the eyebrows and is commonly known as the third eye. Within the symbolic representation of the Ajna center is the syllable *Ohm* which represents the beginning and end of all things. It is from this center that a person harmonizes the forces within him/herself and achieves a balance between Yin and Yang. As the Ajna center is awakened, reunion becomes complete and a person experiences him/herself in the fullness as the I AM, the union of selves.

The third eye radiates a deep blue which in the developed personality borders on violet. It functions as the central point where different flows of Prana meet and are distributed. (Sushumna branches through it, and the Ida and Pingala go right through it after they branch off to the nostrils.) The chakra has control over seeing, not only in the physical sense but in the mystical sense of seeing into the higher planes; intuitive seeing, clairvoyance and the other paranormal forms of knowing. It is the seat of creativity, and when active and open, the seat of Divine Intelligence. The Ajna center controls all higher mental activities. This includes intuitive thought, rational thought and memory. Intuitive thought includes all forms of paranormal activity.

When the student has activated the third eye, he can go beyond merely sensing energy fields and atmospheres. He becomes capable of seeing clairvoyantly, communicating telepathically and healing through mental projection. Also, through the power of his own mind, he can create new realities for himself on the physical plane. The objective reality we experience in the physical world is the physical manifestation of the subject reality created beforehand on the mental plane. Before the sixth chakra becomes active, the process is largely an unconscious one. For persons who have activated their sixth chakra, the process becomes completely conscious and by the power of their own will and imagination, they can create new realities for themselves which conform of their Dharma and speed them toward their goal of wholeness and unconditional joy.

A person who has activated the sixth chakra goes beyond earthly goals and the earthly attachments which divert most people from fulfilling their Dharma. A person who has awakened the Ajna center experiences the new realities created mentally, being transmuted into physical reality, without delay.

When the sixth chakra is opened, consciousness and unconsciousness merge and whatever gulf there was beforehand is permanently abolished. Integration becomes complete and a person sees himself as the union of selves, the I AM. A person in this condition remembers and experiences himself at every stage of his life from the cradle upwards, and he remembers all those individual energy fields that combined to create his particular energy field, including those two most important fields "mother and father." Because his remembrance is complete, he can go beyond the point of terror, beyond the moment he first experienced separation from the universal field to a time when there was only union and unconditional love. In this way, a person becomes his own mother and his own father.

Hermann Hesse intuitively understood this when he wrote that Siddharta ". . . bent over the water . . . he saw his face reflected, and there was something in this reflection that reminded him of something he had forgotten and when he reflected on it he remembered. His face resembled that of another person, whom he had once known, loved and even feared. It resembled the face of his father, the Brahman."[9]

Ajna Meditation

In the Ajna meditation, you will get in touch with the quality which harmonizes everything within you. To begin the Ajna meditation, find a comfortable position with your back straight. Close your eyes and begin breathing yogically. Breathe deeply through your nose without separation between inhalation and exhalation, and feel yourself relaxing. Take your time and become conscious of your body by following your breath for about five minutes. After five minutes, bring your attention to your sixth chakra, between your eyebrows. Then bring your breath to your sixth chakra. On each inhalation feel the energy centered in your third eye grow stronger. You will feel it as a heat and intensity which will grow stronger on each inhalation.

As it grows more powerful, visualize the energy there as a ball of indigo light. Experience and visualize it growing stronger and brighter for about two or three minutes. Then feel your consciousness move upward until it reaches a point between your eyebrows and feel your consciousness centered in the ball of energy. Then become the ball of energy and feel yourself radiating from that center through your body and into the outer environment.

Feel yourself as the union of selves. Feel your mind radiate in all directions simultaneously and feel yourself fill the room with your consciousness. Pay attention to how you feel physically, emotionally and mentally. The more you are centered in the third eye, the more complete will be the union between consciousness and unconsciousness. In this condition you will feel what seems like an electrical current running through your physical body, and your entire head will begin to glow with the center of this fire being the third eye.

Take at least ten minutes for this part of the meditation. After ten minutes, or when you are satisfied, take a deep breath through your nose and as you exhale mentally repeat,

"Every time I come to this level of consciousness, I learn to use more of my mind in more creative ways." Then let your breathing return to normal, release the ball of energy by your sixth chakra and the imagery associated with it and mentally return to the room and relax. After a few moments begin to count mentally from one to five and when you reach the number five, open your eyes. You will feel wide awake, perfectly relaxed and better than you did before.

The Sahasrara Chakra

The seventh chakra is called *Sahasrara* in Sanskrit. It is most often described in the Yogic texts as a thousand-petaled lotus. Some texts locate the chakra at the crown of the head, while other texts declare that it is located above the crown of the head in order to differentiate it from the other six. By awakening the Ajna center, a person has achieved wholeness through the process of psychospiritual integration. He has transcended fear, identified himself as the I AM, and experienced unconditional joy. His development is not complete because although he knows himself in his multiplicity, his experience of self is still differentiated from the All. There is still duality. The final step which is the merging of a person's personal energy field with the universal field (the merging of the I AM with the All), only takes place when the thousand-petaled lotus blossoms and the Kundalini arrives and fully awakens Sahasrara.

Subject, object and God
The Inspirer of the Both
All three are (formed in) Brahma
And nothing but Brahma.
Knowing this one should try to realize HIM in
one's own Being.
Nothing remains to be known after this.[10]

In Tantra, the awakening of the crown chakra corresponds to the union of Shakti (the feminine principle) with Shiva (the masculine principle). This union, once formed, lasts forever. By achieving this state, a person goes beyond the confines of sequential time and finds himself centered always in the unchanging eternal present. He goes beyond the state where he chooses self unconsciously at every moment to the state where self doesn't exist, where self becomes the entire universe which is contained within it. By being the universe, the person ceases to understand his universe because to understand is to cease to be.

Shih-ton, a Zen master, was asked a question by one of his students concerning Dharma. He answered, "Ask the post over there." The student replied, "I do not understand" to which Shih-ton replied, "Neither do I."[11]

When the Ajna center is awakened, a person experiences reunion with the All and everything contained in the All. There is no return from this state. There is no death when this state is achieved. There is nothing but emptiness, and in emptiness one finds himself in the All, the universal field of energy and consciousness.

In the Tao te Ching it is written:

I do my utmost to attain emptiness
I hold firmly to stillness
The myriad creatures all rise together
And I watch them return.
The teaming creatures
All return to their separate roots.
Returning to one's roots is known as stillness.
This is what is meant by returning to one's
    destiny.
Returning to one's destiny is known as the
    constant.
Knowledge of the constant is known as

discernment
Woe to him who willfully innovates
While ignorant of the constant
But should one act from knowledge of the
   constant
One's action will lead to impartiality
Impartiality to kingliness
Kingliness to heaven.
Heaven to the Way.[12]

The crown chakra corresponds to the pineal gland which glows with a violet color when awakened. It is the last chakra to be awakened and therefore corresponds to the highest level of spiritual perfection. Like the other chakras, it is a channel for higher energies—in this case from the causal plane. However, unlike the others, when fully active it can reverse itself and then it radiates like a central sun creating energy and forming above the head of the individual a veritable crown of pure light and divine energy.[13]

Sahasrara Meditation

When it comes to the crown chakra, no meditation is possible because a person doesn't exist as a separate being any longer but instead at every moment he is in union with the All and the All at every moment is meditating through him.

Sitting quietly, doing nothing
Spring comes, and the grass grows by itself[14]

CHAPTER XIII

CHAKRA THERAPY

The real meaning of human existence is to make
manifest in the world the Divine Being embodied
within us, then the true significance and bodily
training lies in the need to reach a state that
makes such manifestation possible.
—Karlfreid Durckheim
The Way of Transformation

There are only four basic emotions from which all other
emotions are built: joy, anger, pain and fear. There is no
negativity inherent in any of them. It is by combining these
basic emotions and applying them to specific situations that
the whole host of other emotions are formed.

The emotions of anger, pain and fear aren't in themselves negative, and they don't feel negative when they are
permitted their natural expression—when they are not
blocked by contraction as they travel through the subtle
energy system. It is these reservoirs of blocked emotions
which feel bad. In truth, anger, pain and fear are merely the
names we give to different frequencies of Prana which flow
through the subtle energy system. In psychospiritual integration, we recognize that all energy is good energy. Problems with energy only arise when through overload or block-

age we have energy at the wrong place at the wrong time.

Like little children we should have no fear in expressing our feelings honestly in all circumstances whatsoever, and we should feel no remorse afterwards for doing so. As long as the emotions are being expressed spontaneously (honestly and courageously), there will be no damage to the subtle energy system and thereby nothing negative will be experienced when the frequencies of energy (emotions) are being expressed.

However, through the process of acculturation, people have learned to block the free radiation of energy, in particular emotional energy, through the subtle energy system. In this way, people have created "others" within themselves and they carry the "others" within them throughout their lives. People's unconscious goals and attitudes, and in many cases their conscious goals and attitudes, reflect their early education and the number and power of the "others" buried within them.

The inner self seeks to express itself and to radiate spontaneously in all circumstances. There is never a question of whether self-expression is good or bad. To be human, it is appropriate to express oneself spontaneously.

If people expressed their emotions spontaneously, which means at the appropriate time with an economy of energy, people would not have any problems with their emotions. It is not the energy or the movement of energy which hurts, rather it is the lack of movement which causes pressure within the subtle energy system, and it is the pressure caused by too much energy being stuck for too long in the wrong place which makes us hurt.

Safety Valves

As long as we live in this world, the chakras act as pressure valves for the subtle energy system. By being open, they prevent an unhealthy build-up of energy within it and they allow emotions to flow through the system naturally. It is essential that the valves stay open and unblocked so that energy is allowed to flow through them, otherwise dangerous pressures develop and the system which the valves are designed to protect will overload and break down after a while.

Unfortunately, people have been taught from infancy to disrupt the natural function of the chakras by altering their natural behavior so that their behavior would conform to social norms. In spite of their best intentions, each generation has unconsciously succeeded in causing their children suffering by forcing them to block the free expression of emotional energy, i.e. Prana, through their subtle energy system. Since it is primarily through the chakras that Prana radiates into the outer environment, any effort to restrict the flow of emotions will, in effect, constrict all frequencies of Prana at their points of entrance, exit and transfer. As pressure increases in the subtle energy system because of the build-up of blocked energy, the chakras close down. The physical body becomes deadened and a person becomes numb. This combination of fear, blockage, pressure and more fear first disrupts the subtle energy system, but soon this disruption is transmuted in all directions until it disrupts a person's life on all four levels of causation.

Notwithstanding earlier damage to the chakras caused by blockages in the subtle energy system, it is possible to heal them and recover the chakras' full function. In this chapter you will find a series of exercises designed to repair the damage by opening your chakras, balancing them and releasing reservoirs of blocked energy caused by the blockages.

Physical Relaxation
The next series of exercises are designed to improve the flow of energy through your subtle energy system.

Their effect is gradual, and because of this they are meant to be done regularly. They are not designed for crisis intervention or for breaking down blockages. Rather they gradually open the chakras, wear blockages away and help your physical body and subtle energy system remember their original state of wholeness, balance and unconditional joy.

The three groups of exercises below are meant to be done one after the other. Their effect is cumulative. Each exercise will get you ready for the next. The first exercise is designed to prepare your physical body for an increased flow of Prana by releasing muscle tension.

Begin by lying on your back, head directly between your shoulders, with your eyes closed. Your legs should be stretched out straight in front of you, hands by your sides. In order to achieve a sense of limpness and abandon necessary for complete physical relaxation, begin by raising your right leg about two inches off the floor. Without a break in the movement, let it drop again as though it were an inanimate object. Next, raise your left leg and without a break in the movement, let it drop.

In the same way raise your right arm slightly and let it drop. Then raise your left arm slightly and let it drop. Next, raise your left leg and right arm together and let them drop simultaneously. Follow this by raising your right leg and left arm together, and without a break in the movement, let them drop simultaneously. Next raise your hips slightly and let them drop. Then raise your chest slightly and let it drop. Finally, roll your head slightly from side to side. These simple movements should make you feel as limp as a rag doll.

For the next few moments lie absolutely still and pay attention to how you feel. Notice how your muscles, tendons, joints, spine and nervous system are readjusting themselves.

As your physical body relaxes, pay attention to the

rhythm of your breath. Feel it get deeper and slower until it seems to be suspended completely. Soon you will begin to experience a sense of weightlessness. You will feel as though your physical body has been transformed into pure energy. Feel this energy revitalize and recharge every molecule of your body. Take about five minutes to relax in the same position. By practicing this relaxation exercise, you will find it easier to succeed with the next group of exercises.

After you have finished the introductory exercise above, you will be ready to proceed with the yogic locks.

Locks

The ancient Yogis created a series of three exercises they called *locks*. These exercises were designed to facilitate the flow of energy through the chakras. However, the regular practice of these locks has a beneficial and rejuvenating effect on the whole subtle energy system as well as the nervous system and physical body.

It is best to do all three locks either lying on your back with your hands at your sides, in the lotus position, or sitting in a straight back chair with your legs in front of you, placed firmly on the floor. Your back should be straight while you are doing all of these locks. Your eyes should be closed and you should be breathing yogically.

The Neck Lock

The *Jalandhara Bandha* or neck lock is the first lock the student should master. It releases energy (particularly Yang energy traveling up the back) which tends to be blocked in the region of the upper chest, shoulders and neck. (Fourth and fifth chakra.) Perform the lock as you inhale through your nose.

Begin by pulling your chin in and contracting your neck so that you feel like you are squeezing them together. At the same time, pull your shoulders up so that the back of your head is resting on your shoulder muscles. It will feel a little like you have no neck at all. Keep your head centered and don't tilt it forward or backward. Once you have achieved the lock, bring your attention to your spine just below your neck and you will feel a tingling sensation radiating from that point upward along the spine into your neck. As it moves upward it will grow stronger and will radiate in all directions. Some people feel a heat accompanying the tingling sensation or even a strong vibration. All of these sensations are normal. Don't do anything to disrupt them or enhance them. Just observe them. The sensations are symptomatic of an increased, healthier flow of Prana up the spine and through the throat chakra.

When you first begin using the lock, I suggest you hold it for a count of five while at the same time you retain your breath. After the count of five, exhale and release the lock. Then rest for a count of five. Repeat for another count of five, then rest. Then do the lock for a third time. After you have finished the third repetition, rest for about two minutes while breathing yogically, until you feel that the energy is flowing smoothly up the back of your neck. When it is flowing without restriction, you will be feeling a glowing sensation in the back of your neck and shoulders which will be accompanied by a feeling of self-contained confidence and inner strength.

The Jalandhara Bandha is important physically because it straightens the upper spine so that Prana is permitted free passage past the throat chakra upward through the sixth and seventh chakra. It benefits the physical body by breaking up tension in the back of the neck and shoulders. It will help you improve your posture and will stimulate the normal physical sensations in this region of your body. The thyroid as well as parathyroid glands are stimulated by the pressure put on them, and this helps them to secrete hormones more efficiently. By functioning optimally, the higher

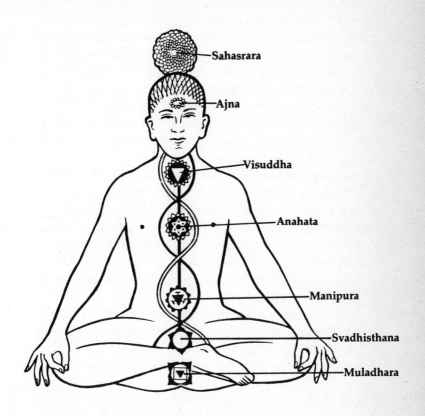

Sahasrara

Ajna

Visuddha

Anahata

Manipura

Svadhisthana

Muladhara

The Seven Chakras

functions of the pituitary and pineal glands are enhanced.

In dealing with the energy moving past the heart and throat chakra (in particular the heart chakra), we are dealing with a combination of energies. These energies differ in polarity. On one side we have Yin, which is feminine, and on the other side Yang, which is masculine. As Yin and Yang energy enter the field of each chakra, the chakra exerts a certain pulling force like gravity on the energy.

When there is a preponderence of Yin energy going through a chakra, as it passes down the front of the body through the great conceptual (feminine) channel, then a person's physical condition, and for that matter his subtle energy system, will be more receptive or passive. When there is a preponderence of Yang energy going through the chakra, as it travels up the back through the governor (masculine) channel, there will be a preponderence of masculine assertive energy in the physical and subtle bodies and subtle energy system, and the person will be overly assertive and nonreceptive.

The importance of the neck lock lies in its ability to correct imbalances in the mixture of Yin and Yang energy as it flows in, out and past the fourth and fifth chakra. It does this by breaking up tension in the physical body which restricts the flow of energy through either the conceptual or governor meridian. A restriction in either channel can cause a host of energy problems from depression to hyperactivity depending on the balance between Yin and Yang. When the conceptual channel is restricted, then the symptoms tend toward arrogance and hyperactivity. When the governor is restricted, the symptoms tend toward passivity and depression.

The Diaphragm Lock

The Yddiyana Bandha or diaphragm lock is the second lock. You begin the lock by lifting your diaphragm up in the direction of the chest cavity while you pull the organs of the upper abdomen up and back toward the spine. This lock should only be applied on the exhalation, in order to make room in the chest cavity for the contraction.

Begin by holding the lock for a count of five and bring your attention to the middle of your back behind the solar plexus while you retain your breath. After a few moments you will feel a tingling sensation beginning in your back directly behind the solar plexus. The sensation will grow in intensity until it widens into a warm glow which will travel up the spine toward the heart chakra. As it flows upward, some of this energy will be forced through the third chakra by the chakra's natural magnetic pull. The subtle energy system will use this energy which the chakra transmutes in order to increase a person's sense of belonging, contentment, as well as to improve relationships. After you have held the lock for a count of five, release it as you inhale for a count of five. Repeat the lock three times; after the third repetition, relax while you continue breathing yogically for about five minutes and pay attention to the energy flowing up through your third chakra.

The Yddiyana Bandha is particularly helpful for developing empathy and compassion since it stimulates the flow of energy through and past the solar plexus chakra. This can be a crucial lock for those people who have difficulty in connecting with people and maintaining long-term relationships. By stimulating the solar plexus, in effect it stimulates the entire sympathetic nervous system. Stimulating the sympathetic nervous system promotes the flow of nervous energy which furthers the processes of nutrition, assimilation and growth. Further, there is no completely emotional satisfying experience possible, or for that matter, emotional release possible, without the physical body being involved. The physical body is under the direct control of the sympathetic nervous system, so by stimulating the third chakra, a person stimulates those centers of awareness which permit

the expression .of emotional energy completely through
the physical body.

The Root Lock

The third lock is the *Mulabandha* or root lock. It is the
most complex. Its importance for us lies primarily in the
powerful effect on Kundalini stored at the base of the spine
and the sexual energy of the second chakra. In the first part
of the root lock you must contract the anal sphincter and
draw it in, the same way you would to hold in a bowel
movement; then pull in the sexual organs so that there is a
contraction along the urinary tract and in the lower trunk.
In the final part, you draw in the lower abdomen at the
navel point, pulling it back toward the spine. This draws the
rectum and sexual organs up and back toward the back.

This lock should be done on exhalation and should be
held for a count of five, then released for a count of five, and
repeated three times. After the third time, relax the body,
breathe yogically and rest for five minutes or for as long as
you feel comfortable, paying attention to the flow of energy
in the lower and upper abdomen, and along the lower
spine.

This lock releases blockages in the first and second
chakra thereby stimulating sexual and creative energy as
well as stimulating the release of Kundalini which lies dormant at the base of the spine.

As you progress, there is a variation of this exercise
you can do which is beneficial. You should only attempt it
after you have mastered the individual locks.

Begin the variation by sitting on your heels with your
hands on your thighs, close your eyes and begin breathing
yogically. After two or three minutes, apply the root lock.
Relax it without holding it. Then apply the diaphragm lock
and relax it without holding it. Finally apply the neck lock
and relax it without holding it. Repeat the three locks in this

order rhythmically for three or four minutes. Your breath will naturally go out on the first two locks and in on the third.

After a few moments your physical body will sweat and it will begin releasing toxins. This is a cleansing for the physical body and is very useful because the physical body, when obstructed in any way, will inhibit the free flow of Prana through the subtle energy system. Doing the locks from the bottom up also helps to awaken the Kundalini and promotes its flow upward toward the crown chakra. As you become stronger, you can increase the length of time you do the exercises—from three to four minutes to as long as ten minutes. It is important, however, to never strain. Listen to your body and intuition, and stop when they tell you to. Straining does nothing to help your energy system. In truth, it is very dangerous and can lead to grave difficulties.

Opening and Balancing the Chakras

The third exercise is called Chakra Balancing. It enhances the flow of energy passing through the chakras.

Chakra balancing in combination of the first two groups of exercises in this chapter will enhance your ability to radiate energy freely.

You should begin chakra balancing from the same position you were in when you finished the locks. It makes no difference if you sit or lie down. Just make sure your back is straight. Your eyes should be closed and you should be relaxed.

Begin counting backwards from five to one, and on each descending number take a long deep breath and feel yourself getting more and more relaxed. There is no need to control the mind in any way, but simply let it go where it likes. When you have reached the number one, silently repeat the affirmation, "I am deeply relaxed, feeling better than I did before."

Then pay attention to the first chakra, which is at the base of your spine. As soon as you pay attention to it, the chakra will begin to vibrate and tingle. That is how you can locate each chakra, the tingling sensation originates from its center. By paying attention to your chakras, you will experience them opening and expanding. You can feel the very spot where they are located and the pulsating tingling sensation caused by the energies passing through them into your aura.

By paying attention to the first chakra, not only can you locate it, but the mental force of your attention serves to activate it. This mental stimulation is the first step in opening the chakras. The next step is breathing from each individual chakra. In this way you can stimulate them even further by bringing the energy inherent in the breath which is a manifestation of Prana (the vital force) to the chakras. With these two tools, the mind and the breath, at your service, you can easily initiate the process of opening and balancing your energy centers. Begin at the first chakra (base of the spine) by mentally paying attention to it. Next breathe into it, and then without separation between inhalation and exhalation, breathe out, and as you do chant the universal *Ohm* from the chakra.

The important thing to remember in the last stage (chanting on the exhalation) is that the musical note you chant must cause a sympathetic vibration in the chakra in the same way a sympathetic vibration is caused in a violin string when a tuning fork which has the same tone is struck next to it. Repeat the process of chanting *Ohm* three times from each chakra, starting at the base of the spine and ending at the crown.

Raise the *Ohm* one note for each chakra, beginning with G for the first chakra, going through the seven notes of the scale (as you go through the seven chakras).

After you have chanted three times from each chakra,

remain in the same position with your eyes closed for about five minutes. Breathe yogically and pay attention to how you feel physically, emotionally and mentally. After five minutes, or when you feel satisfied, mentally count from one to five. When you reach the number five, open your eyes. You will feel wide awake, perfectly relaxed and better than you did before.

The combination of techniques, physical relaxation, the locks and chakra balancing takes only about 15 minutes, but even though they take such a short time their combined effects can be remarkable. Not only are the chakras opened, but they are balanced, creating a healthy flow of energy in the subtle energy system. This in turn strengthens and revitalizes the physical body and nervous system, and this will safeguard each one of you from negativity encountered in both the internal and external environment.

These techniques should ideally be practiced every day, in the morning or late afternoon. I do not recommend practicing them around bedtime, since they tend to stimulate the nerves and can keep you awake. If you practice them regularly you will soon begin to experience their effects. Your mind will become more alert and you will experience less internal dialogue. Anxiety will decrease and you will feel more relaxed and emotionally open. Furthermore, your energy level will increase, filling you with a greater sense of well-being.

The exercises, by releasing old reservoirs of energy and stimulating the flow of energy through your subtle energy system, enable you to remember and recollect yourself and help you to achieve wholeness and unconditional joy.

CHAPTER XIV

PRANA AND CHAKRA CLEANSING

When the light of knowledge gleams forth from
all the gates of the body, then be sure that
purity prevails.

—*Bhagavad Gita*

Prana in Sanskrit means the absolute energy. It is the
original source of all forms of energy found in our multi-
dimensional universe. Prana, in combination with consciousness, mysteriously becomes life. When this life force combines
with matter we have the myriad of life forms which inhabit
the manifest physical universe. The level of consciousness
of a particular life form is dependent on the frequencies of
Prana that it can channel and store in its subtle energy system. Animals are animated by a much lower range of frequencies than man, and spiritual man by a much higher range of
frequencies than primitive man. There are fluctuations in the
consciousness of all living things based on a fluctuation in the
range of energy frequencies traveling through the system, but
the fluctuations cannot exceed the capabilities of the chakras
and nadis to conduct them and the auras to store them.

Auras
The auras are reservoirs of subtle energy. Each aura is a

reservoir for a specific range of frequencies. It is thought that the word aura comes from the Sanskrit root *ar* which means spokes (like the spokes of a wheel). Conceptually, the aura could be considered a radiation coming from a specific point. It is sometimes described as a radiation of Prana or vital force which is common to all life forms.

Viewed in this way, the aura of a particular being can be thought of as a subtle emanation or extension of a sub-field within the entities' personal energy field. The aura is an extension of the personal energy field of any creature which radiates beyond the centers of consciousness within the personal energy field of the creature. One can liken the aura to the atmosphere surrounding the Earth. The atmosphere is not the Earth itself, but it has an intimate relationship to the Earth, influences it and is influenced by it. The atmosphere extends far beyond the planet, becoming finer the further away it is. It is a buffer between the outer environment, space and the planet itself. The auras extend beyond the physical and subtle bodies like an atmosphere, and like an atmosphere they serve as buffers between a person and the outer environment.

The influence of the auras over a person's well-being should not be underestimated. It is essential that the auras are healthy and in balance with one another in order to secure the health of the subtle energy system, and a healthy interaction between an individual and his outer environment.

An understanding of the auras and their function can be seen in many cultures over many thousands of years. In Babylon, ancient Egypt, China, India, Israel and Greece as well as most if not all tribal traditions, human radiations and the aura specifically were acknowledged and represented symbolically. We can see this representation in the head-dress of Egyptian priests, in the auras around the early Saints and in the representatives of the Great Buddha. The Druids believed in and symbolically poured auric fluid into their jewelry during casting to provide the wearer more of this vital substance.

It was believed by the ancients that the aura was an emanation of the blood. In the symbolic drinking of Christ's blood during Communion we have the symbolic merging of the devotees' auric field with the auric field of Christ. The Bible makes many other references to the auric field. When Moses came down from Mount Sinai we are told that His face shone and the Israelites were unable to gaze upon it. St. Steven, the first Christian martyr, began to glow, his face becoming radiant as he was being stoned for his beliefs.

Most authorities agree that there are three auras. The spiritual aura is a reservoir of spiritual energy which surrounds a person. It is egg-shaped and extends equally in all directions about 26 feet around a person. The mental aura is a reservoir of mental energy which surrounds a person. It is egg-shaped and extends about eight feet in all directions. The etheric aura is a reservoir of energy from the astral body, the etheric double and physical body. Like the spiritual and mental auras, it is egg-shaped and surrounds a person. It extends about eight inches around a person in all directions. An important property of the etheric aura is that the energy within it pulsates and can be affected by the breath. Because of this property, a person can positively influence the condition of their etheric aura by breathing yogically.

Every person has a personal aura which is a combination of spiritual, mental and etheric auras. The personal auras of groups or crowds can combine with one another, and if there is one dominant mood or feeling, a collective group aura will be created as they come together. This collective aura can be experienced in cities or any area where people are crowded together. The collective aura created by a group will have a powerful effect on any person caught within it, often sweeping him into the collective energy field, in a sense manipulating him to participate energetically and mentally with the group.

In groups that come together to share devotion or love, this collective aura can so intensify the prevailing field that people are swept into much higher energy levels and states of consciousness than normal. On the other hand, in a mob stirred by mass feeling, a person will have to exert great force in order to resist the combined mental and emotional pull of the negative field and to keep his aura free from contamination.

Attraction and Rejection

The ability to connect with a person to experience him energetically by sensing the energy fields that surround him is an innate inability of all human beings. When energy fields are primarily experienced on the unconscious level, they are often experienced as a vague positive or negative feeling which makes you feel good or bad about somebody. The energy field surrounding a person which is the combined field created by their spiritual, mental and etheric auras has a great influence on whether we like him, feel comfortable with him or trust him. In dealing with other people, we judge them far more for how they feel to us than for what they do for us. People are drawn to other people whose auras resonate in the same way as their own, and no matter how a person disguises himself by his actions or appearance, his energy field will give him away and he will be recognized by someone whose personal energy field resonates in the same range of frequencies.

Research into human energy fields has shown that when the mental and etheric auras of people who like each other come in contact there is a blending of the fields. They flow into one another, imbuing both parties with a deep feeling of belonging which can lead them into an experience of union.

Morphogenetic Fields

Work by scientists, such as Rupert Sheldrake, is suggesting a scientific explanation for human behavior and interaction based on energy fields and the human aura. Mr. Sheldrake calls energy fields, in particular human energy fields, morphogenetic fields. In his Theory of Formative Causation he postulates that all life forms from viruses through human beings derive their structure not solely from DNA or known physical causes but from the influence of past forms (fields). Sheldrake calls this influence morphogenetic (from the Greek words *morpho* which means "form" and *genesis* which means "beginning") fields.

According to Sheldrake, the form and development not only of living beings but of matter (such as the formation of crystals) are shaped and maintained by morphogenetic fields. These fields overlap, but they work on the like-influence-like principle. Fields for humans for example, have little effects on rats. Life forms come under the influence of morphogenetic fields through a phenomenon Sheldrake calls morphic resonance, a kind of tuning into past life forms. Morphic resonance works across both time and space.

Thus, a stalk of corn takes up its characteristic shape and form not because its DNA commands it, but because it participates in the same fields that all the corn stalks that preceded it participated in. This field guides it through its development through morphic resonance. Sheldrake describes the process as "a kind of connective memory between species to which all members contribute and from which all members draw upon."

He believes there is a hierarchy of morphogenetic fields. For the human organism there would be a field which guides the development of cells, another field over that one for individual tissues such as the heart and liver, one over that for the entire human body as a whole. Finally, he suggests that interpenetrating all these individual fields is a universal morphogenetic field from which the patterns for all life forms come.

Taking this idea even further, Sheldrake also theorizes the existence of morphogenetic fields influencing (though not controlling) behavior and thought. Once a species picks up a particular habit or idea, it becomes part of the morphogenetic field for that species. As a result it becomes easier for later generations to learn a particular behavior, even for members of the species who had no physical contact with earlier generations who previously learned the new behavior. They simply pick it up if circumstances or environment cause them to tune in to that part of the field.

When Sheldrake began looking for evidence for morphic resonance, he began plowing through the voluminous literature on animal behavior tested in labs. He knew that if he was correct, a rat learning a trick in a lab in one part of the world should make it easier for a rat in a laboratory in another part of the world to learn the same trick.

Sheldrake was worried at first because it seemed that if this presumption was true, it should have been noticed already. He almost gave up on the idea before realizing the evidence might be there but no one recognized it. He eventually landed on a series of experiments begun in 1920 at Harvard by a W. McDougall, who was trying to prove a hypothesis somewhat different from Sheldrake's: that knowledge was passed from parents to children genetically.

McDougall conducted his experiment on 32 generations of white rats. Each rat was placed in a tub of water. Escape was through one of two gangways. One brightly lit path gave the rat an electric shock when it passed through and the other, a dimly lit one, did not. The first generation of rats learned very slowly with an average of 56 mistakes per rat, but their descendants made fewer and fewer mistakes with each generation, and the last group tested averaged 20 mistakes. The same curve appeared for descendants of the slowest learning rats as well as the smart ones, and many of the rats of the later generations demonstrated more caution and hesitation in their reactions. Some kind of untaught knowledge seemed to be evident.

Recently, psychologist Arden Mahlberg of Midwestern Psychological Services in Madison, Wisconsin, added some credibility to Sheldrake's hypothesis with a unique experiment.

He presented students with a speed-learning test of International Morse code and a second test of a novel code composed of the same symbols. He divided the students into several groups and tested each group at a different time.

Morse code, as it turned out, was easier to learn for the first group. The novel code, as would be expected if morphogenetic fields exist, was more difficult to learn than Morse. It became easier to learn, however, as it was learned by increasing numbers of students and was actually easier to learn than Morse for the last group. "Both codes," said Mahlberg, "showed evidence of Sheldrake's phenomenon."

Brain Mind Connection

Recent research into the nature of thought and the relationship between the brain and mind have led to new scientific insights which seem to validate the fact that energetic fields in particular for mind and thought exist.

Karl Pribram, a scientist at Stanford University, began studying the relationship between the brain and mind at the Yerkes Laboratory of Primate Biology in 1946 where Karl Lashley, a physiological psychologist, was working. Lashley was cutting slices out of rats' brains to see whether he could trace particular memories-memory traces, or engrams to particular parts of the cerbral cortex. But when his trained rats still performed learned tasks with large amounts

of their brain tissue removed, Lashley put forth the unortho-
dox notion that memory is somehow distributed throughout
the brain.

This brought up fundamental questions such as, where
is consciousness encoded in the physical brain? Or, is "mind"
something outside the physical brain, is it something non-
physical and spiritual?

By the late 1960's, questions such as these had co-
alesced for Pribram into his holographic model of the brain.
What Pribram proposed is that the brain stores information
via mathematical codes similar to those used in holography, a
lensless photographic process invented by Dennis Gabor
in 1947.

Unlike an ordinary photograph, which is a two-
dimensional image of an object, a hologram is a lifelike
three-dimensional image formed by light. Its stored code
on film doesn't look anything like the visual image; rather it
is a record of the wave patterns scattered by the object.
Imagine dropping two pebbles into a pond and freezing the
surface immediately so that the frozen overlapping ripple
patterns record the pebbles' passage through a moment of
time. That's how a hologram works. A beam of light energy—
a laser, in most cases—is split in two, one part traveling
directly to the holographic film as a reference beam, while
the other is first bounced off the object to be photographed.
The two beams then collide on the film, which stores the
interference pattern of the two intersecting wavefronts: the
pristine, undisturbed reference and its twin beam that has
been "disturbed" by the object. It's this "disturbance" that
the hologram records, though on the actual film all one can
see is an apparently meaningless pattern of dark and light
swirls. But when illuminated by a reconstruction beam, a
three-dimensional image results. It's as if the object's wavefront had been frozen in time in the holographic plate until
the beam releases it to continue its path to your eye.

It is in this way Pribram theorizes that memories and images are stored in our brains. Perhaps when we recall something particular, Pribram suggests, we're using a specific "reconstruction beam" to zoom in on a particular encoded memory. He also fixes upon another quality of the hologram: the fact that it records the same wavefront across its entire surface, repeating it over and over. Should you drop and shatter a hologram and salvage only a fragment of the plate, it will still be enough to reconstruct the entire image. Pribram feels that the brain's scattered code likewise allows memories to survive sometimes awesome damage. He theorizes that what we call mind may be stored in the physical brain as a sort of ghostly hologram—located everywhere and nowhere at the same time.

In an interview in 1982, Pribram was asked whether the mind could be part of a universal whole, a universal field. He answered: "The world is not a hologram, only one aspect, one order, is holographic. But the holographic domain is holistic in a different sense from the Gestalt use of the word. In Gestalt, the whole is greater than, and different from, the sum of its parts, whereas in a hologram, every part is distributed in the whole, and the whole is enfolded in its parts. David Bohm (professor of theoretical physics at Birkbeck College in London, and author of "Wholeness and the Implicate Order") has derived the same idea from quantum physics and it leads to a scientific understanding of the spiritual aspects of man's experience. For the first time in three hundred years, science is admitting spiritual values into its explorations."[1]

The Egg

The health of a person's personal energy field (the auras) and its ability to interact in a healthy way with other energy fields is so important for us in psychospiritual integration that we cannot leave it to chance that the auras remain healthy and strong. We must ensure that our auras can store and distribute energy properly and that energy can flow in and out from them freely. Moreover, our auras must be able to transmute unhealthy frequencies of energy into healthy ones. In order to promote the health and balance of the auras and their sensitivity to outside fields, I have designed a technique called the "Egg."

The Egg has a powerful effect on the subtle energy system, in particular the auras. It strengthens them and helps them to retain their integrity, especially when they come into contact with fields which would ordinarily disrupt them. The strength and integrity of the auras depend on the quality and quantity of energy within them as well as their pressure. The pressure of energy within a person's individual auras is important because it determines the relationship each aura has with the ones adjacent to it. Pressure within the auras is determined by the amount of Prana in the auras, and the chakras' ability to transmute frequencies of energy entering and exiting the auras efficiently and quickly. Pressure must be considered because it has an important influence on the overall strength of the auric fields surrounding the body.

The first serious sign that there has been a disruption of energy pressure in the auras is a breakdown of will. We can look at will as energy dependent. The more integrity within the subtle energy system, i.e. the fewer blockages and the stronger and more consistent the pressure, the stronger and more consistent a person's will power. The access outside energy has to a person's energy system, its ability to enter an auric field and to transmute frequencies of energy within it is directly related to a person's will power. In other words, we cannot think of will as entirely an aspect of the mind but rather an integrated function of our subtle energy system and mental body.

Passivity which is the result of a breakdown of will is

caused by depressurization of the auric fields. It is to strengthen the auras and will power that I have developed the Egg. It will help correct energy problems which have led to a state of passivity. It does this by opening the chakras, promoting the flow of energy through the nadis, and increasing and regulating the pressure in the subtle energy system, especially within the auras.

The Egg is done with a partner. One partner treats the other. The partner taking on the passive role will be called the patient. The partner who is performing the treatment will be called the healer. Imagine that you are the healer in this situation. To begin, find a comfortable room with a good atmosphere which is quiet and where you won't be disturbed. The patient must lie down on the floor, or on a cushion, on the stomach with the hands at the sides. The patient should begin breathing yogically and let his/her mind relax and become quiet. After becoming relaxed and comfortable, the patient puts the tongue to the top of the mouth just behind the teeth to connect the major Yang and Yin streams of energy flowing through his/her subtle energy system.

You as the healer begin the treatment by going into a short meditation which will activate your second attention and open your chakras so that you can be a more effective channel for energy. The simplest way for you to achieve the right level of consciousness is to breathe yogically for a few moments, while sitting on your heels facing the patient's feet. After you feel relaxed, count backward mentally from five to one, mentally repeating and visualizing each number three times. After reaching the number one mentally repeat, "I am now deeply relaxed; every time I come to this level of mind, I learn to go to deeper and healthier levels."

Next you slowly count backward from ten to one, visualizing that on each descending number you're walking down one step of a staircase until you reach the number

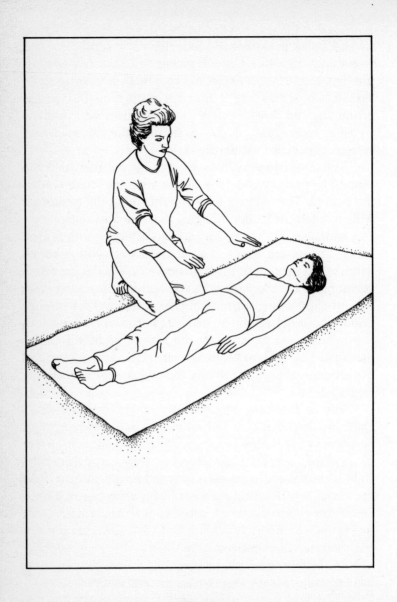

The Egg

one and are at the bottom. When you reach the bottom, you will feel that you are in a much deeper level of consciousness. You will feel weightless, like a feather, so light in fact that you feel like you are beginning to float. At that point you should drift to your perfect place of relaxation. Remain there for two or three minutes and let yourself experience the unconditional joy of your sanctuary.

After two or three minutes, mentally return to the room and affirm to yourself: "I am now in the perfect energy level to work on . . . " and then speak the patient's name. Slowly open your eyes, keeping them slightly unfocused. Next, bring your tongue to the top of your mouth while continuing to breathe yogically. Rub your hands together vigorously for a few moments to polarize them, take a deep breath through the nose and hold your breath. Your palms should be down, horizontal to the floor, fingers comfortably spread apart situated about four inches above the patient's physical body, within his/her etheric aura. Beginning at the patient's feet and with both hands within his/her etheric aura, make a continuous sweep upward from the patient's feet to the top of the head. Then exhale through your mouth. Repeat this part of the exercise six more times for a total of seven sweeps up the patient's body.

After you have completed the sweeps, which is the first part of this three part treatment, begin part two by locating the patient's first chakra. Place your positive hand into the patient's aura at a point just above the patient's first chakra. Next, inhale deeply through the nose. While retaining the breath, begin making counterclockwise circular motions with your hand about two inches above the patient's chakra. Hold your breath for as long as it is comfortable, then exhale through your nose. Without separation between exhalation and inhalation, breathe in again through your nose and retain your breath while rotating your hand

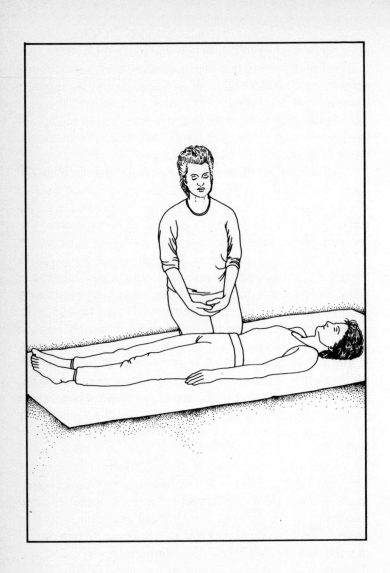

Recharging

again. Breathing in this way increases the flow of Prana between healer and patient, and also enhances your sensitivity
which will make it easier for you to empathize with your
patient.

Continue with the hand movement until you feel em-
pathetically that your patient is taking in the energy that
you are projecting to him/her. When you can sense that
energy is radiating through the patient's first chakra, move
on to the second chakra. Work in the same way all the way
through the patient's seventh chakra.

Have your patient turn over and continue the treatment, working from the patient's sixth chakra down the
front of the patient's body to the first chakra. The only difference as you work down the patient's body is that beginning with the sixth chakra, instead of rotating your hand
counterclockwise, you rotate your hand clockwise. After
you have gone down the front of the patient's body and
have completed the rotating motions over each chakra, you
can begin part three. Part three is identical to part one
except you sweep down the front of your patient's body
from the patient's head to the feet. Make seven sweeps
down the front of the patient's body. After you complete
the seventh sweep, take a few moments to recharge yourself while the patient simply remains in the same position
and enjoys the effects of the treatment.

To recharge yourself, remove your hands from the
patient, sit quietly for a few moments while breathing
yogically. Visualize a wave of energy flowing into your
body through the crown chakra. You should feel the energy
flowing down the back of your spine and then radiating in
every direction, filling your whole body with energy. Recharging in this way should take only two or three minutes.
You will know you are fully recharged when you feel your
higher chakras glowing with energy.

The entire technique—including the time it takes for

recharging—shouldn't take more than 15 minutes, so it can be done easily every day during special times when you or someone close to you feels exhausted, drained, de-pressed or anxious. Depression, exhaustion, anxiety as well as many other conditions are caused by a lack of energy in the personal energy field. The Egg is an excellent treatment which will correct these problems by opening the chakras, promoting the flow of energy through the nadis, and increasing the pressure within the auras by filling them with energy.

CHAPTER XV

NADIS AND THE BREATH OF LIFE

And the Lord God formed man of the dust of the ground, and breathed into his nostrils the breath of life; and man became a living soul.
—*Genesis* 2:7

The word Nadi comes from the root *nad* in Sanskrit and it means hollow stalk. The nadis are channels which carry energy through the subtle energy system. They are inter-dimensional which means they act as arteries carrying vital energy from one subtle body to another. Through the agency of the chakras, the nadis of one subtle body are connected to the nadis of the neighboring bodies. The Varatopanishad tells us that the nadis extend from the bottom of the feet to the top of the head and it is through them that Prana, the "breath of life," flows.

There has been more disagreement over the nadis, what they are and what they do than any other organ of the subtle energy system. Some ancient texts tell us they are identical to the nervous system, while others tell us they correspond to the meridians of acupuncture. We do know that, even with all the disagreement, they are very numerous. One ancient text tells us that 72,000 nadis originate twelve digits above the anus just below the navel in an egg-shaped

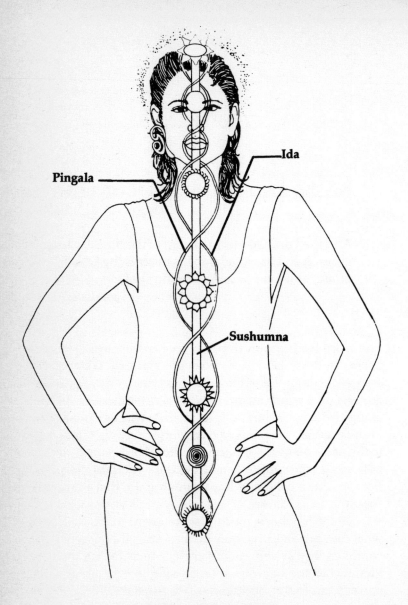

Pingala

Ida

Sushumna

Nadis or Nerve currents

organ called the Kanda (the Kanda seems to correspond to the point the Japanese call Hara). Other texts say there are over 350,000. The disagreements in the ancient texts shouldn't concern us too much because among the thousands of nadis which carry Prana throughout the subtle energy system, there is an essential agreement that there are 72 important nadis and among the 72, ten are of particular concern. Of these, the most vital are: the sushumna, ida and pingala.

The Yogic concept of Nadis gives one description of the system of energy channels while the Chinese and Japanese have a similar system of channels called meridians which form the basis of Chinese medicine.

In the Yogic system it is the sushumna which runs through the center of the spine, beginning at the coccyx and ending at the crown of the head, which is the most important channel. In the Japanese art of Jin Shin Jitsu, sushumna corresponds to the central meridian called the Great Central Channel which is made up of two parts. The conceptual meridian begins at the tongue and runs down the center of the body past the sexual organs to the coccyx where it is connected to the Governor meridian. The Governor follows the same path as the sushumna except that it passes over the head and down past the nose to the top of the mouth. Sushumna is the path of Kundalini (the coiled serpent energy located at the base of the spine) which Yogis consider the most powerful source of energy found in a human being. The Great Central Channel has the same function as it is the main source of Chi energy in the body.

The conceptual meridian is known as "The Great Mother Flow." It is the most important of the Yin meridians. The Governor meridian is the most important of the Yang meridians and is called "The Great Father Flow." In Jin Shin Jitsu, the Great Central Channel is considered to be so important to the well-being of the physical body and subtle energy system that it is considered to be "the ruling energy channel of the body and spirit."[1]

The ancient Yogic texts tell us that the ida and pingala, together with the sushumna, are the ruling nadis and begin at either side of the first chakra (Muladhara). The ida is channeled through the left nostril while the pingala through the right. It is suggested by some authorities that the ida and pingala correspond to the sympathetic nervous system because they are located on either side of the spinal cord. This has never been proven, however. It is much more likely that they correspond to the urinary bladder meridians. Although there are many different schools of thought concerning the nadis in Yoga and the meridians in Chinese medicine, all agree that these channels are passages of vital energy called Chi (Ki) in Chinese medicine and Prana in the Yogic Sutras. The importance of the nadis for us in psychospiritual integration lies in the nadis' two main functions: the first is their ability to absorb Prana directly from the air on inhalation, and their ability to throw off toxins on exhalation. In this function, the nadis can be compared to the blood which takes in oxygen while passing through the lungs on inhalation, and throws off waste products on exhalation.

The second function has to do with activating the serpent energy called Kundalini. The word Kundalini comes from the Sanskrit *Kundala* which means a ring or coil. It is symbolized by a sleeping serpent which faces downward at the base of the sushumna.

In ancient Yogic tradition, we are told that through discipline and exercise a student activates the Kundalini first by having the head of the serpent turn upwards, and then by having it rise through the sushumna until it reaches the crown chakra. When this is accomplished and Kundalini is fully awakened, the ida and pingala merge with the sushumna forming one channel through which this vital force can travel and the student then achieves enlightenment.

To conserve and enhance the flow of energy through the nadis, in particular the ida, pingala and sushumna, and to uncoil the serpent energy lying downwards at the base of sushumna, the ancient Yogis developed a set of breathing exercises called Pranayama. B. K. S. Iyengar tells us that Pranayama " . . . causes the Kundalini to uncoil. The serpent lifts its head, enters the sushumna and is forced up through the chakras one by one to the Sahasrara."[2]

The Bellow's Breath

The exercise below is called the "Bellow's Breath." It is a Pranayama exercise which in Sanskrit is called *Kapalabhati*. *Kapala* means "skull" and *Bhati* means "cleansing the skull." Its main function is to awaken the Kundalini. However, it is also useful in clearing out clogged nadis—in particular the sushumna, pingala and ida. By cleaning them out, Kapalabhati enhances the flow of energy through the subtle energy system. On the physical level, it cleans the nostrils, the ears and the other air passageways inside the head and aids in full oxygenation and removal of toxins from the blood.

The Bellow's Breath is a three-part exercise: rapid expulsion, retention and then slow inhalation. In contrast with normal respiration where inhalation is active and exhalation passive, in Kapalabhati exhalation is active while inhalation is passive. Moreover, in other breathing exercises exhalation is slower than inhalation (generally twice as long). In Kapalabhati, it is the opposite. The Bellow's Breath consists of a sharp exhalation of air in short bursts each of which is followed by a passive inhalation.

When done in moderation, the exercise may be practiced in any position where the back is straight. For now, I suggest you do it either sitting in a straight back chair with the feet flat on the floor and your hands in your lap, or in the lotus position. When you become more advanced, the lotus position is the preferred position. Although we breathe in

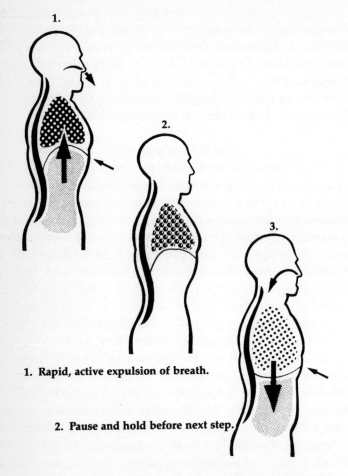

1. Rapid, active expulsion of breath.

2. Pause and hold before next step.

3. Long, slow, passive inhalation of breath.

The Bellow's Breath

and out through the abdomen in the Bellow's Breath, the throat plays an important part in the technique precisely because it stays completely immobile.

To begin the exercise, find a comfortable position with your back straight and begin breathing yogically. Breathe yogically for about two minutes, or until you feel relaxed. Then put your positive hand on your abdomen and for the next few moments pay attention to the rhythm of your breath. Then take a deep breath and fill your abdomen with air. Keep your upper body, especially your chest and throat, straight and rigid. Relax the lower part of your body, in particular the abdomen, so that it is comfortably extended as it fills with air. From this position sharply contract the muscles of your abdomen, especially the large straight ones. This contraction will push the air up and out through your nose. Once the air is expelled, immediately relax the abdomen until it is again slightly extended. Air will naturally be pulled back into your lungs. There is no effort in the inhalation. Then repeat the sharp contraction of your abdominal muscles to force the air up and out again. This is the basic rhythm you must follow in the first part of the exercise.

The first part of the Bellow's Breath consists of a rapid series of sharp rhythmic exhalations followed by passive inhalations. During the passive inhalation, be sure to relax the abdomen gradually so that the air enters relatively slowly. Yogic texts suggest that the expulsion lasts about two-tenths of a second, while the inhalation varies between eight-tenths and three-tenths. However, the speed is not important. Rather it is the rhythm and force of expulsion which gives a person the positive effects of this exercise. You can ensure that the expulsion is optimal by imagining that you are giving a powerful blow to the muscles of the abdomen in the area just below the navel on each exhalation.

The second part of the Bellow's Breath begins right

after your last forced expulsion. After the last forced expulsion, take a long, deep breath through your nose and hold it. At the same time, remove your hand from your abdomen. Retain your breath until you feel a strong surge of energy shooting up your spine from your first chakra through the sushumna to the top of your head, the seventh chakra. As soon as the energy reaches your head, you will feel very lightheaded and even a little dizzy. Immediately exhale through your nose when you feel these sensations. As you exhale, force the Prana which the exercise has released back through your body even while the air is being expelled through your nose.

In this phase of the exercise your breath will be audible like a sigh and it will resemble the breathing of Sumo wrestlers as they prepare themselves to fight. After the first long exhalation, without separation between exhalation and inhalation, take a second breath through your nose.

Continue in this way until your breathing returns to normal. Then take about five minutes to feel the effects that the Bellow's Breath has had on you mentally, emotionally, and physically. After five minutes mentally affirm, "Every time I perform the Bellow's Breath, I strengthen my energy system and bring it back into harmony and balance." Then slowly count mentally from one to five. When you reach the number five, open your eyes. You will feel wide awake, perfectly relaxed and better than you did before.

Kapalabhati can be practiced every day. It is especially good to practice it in the morning before breakfast. When you are doing a series of breathing exercises, it is best to begin with the Bellow's Breath. Don't practice it right after you eat since it will disrupt your digestion, and don't practice it just before you go to sleep since it excites the nerves and subtle energy system and can keep you awake.

The Bellow's Breath is a vigorous exercise. The lungs have to get used to it slowly, and so does the subtle energy system. Since you are increasing both the amount and pressure of Prana flowing through the nadis, it is important not to damage the system by forcing too much energy through a system not strong enough to handle it. During the first week of practice you should carry out groups of 40 exhalations per minute. After the first group, rest for thirty seconds while breathing slowly and easily. Then repeat. Add another ten exhalations to the group each week until finally you reach groups of 100 exhalations per minute, each group of 100 exhalations being followed by a rest period of 30 seconds. Five groups of 100 exhalations are sufficient to achieve the desired results and I suggest you don't go beyond that without more advanced training.

Since this exercise effects the Kundalini, the most powerful stream of energy in the body and is so vigorous, it should be approached with care. Anyone suffering from a lung or bronchial condition should not practice it. Those who suffer from heart trouble should consult a physician before beginning it. Those suffering from emphysema can practice it, since any part that has been permanently affected cannot be made worse by Kapalabhati. However, emphysema indicates that the lungs are very fragile and prudence is required, otherwise further damage is possible.

There are certain common errors that should be avoided by beginning students. Remember that the chest must remain rigid; it does not take part in the exercise. The student should also be careful not to lift the shoulders, pull in the abdomen, or bend the spinal column.

The Positive Effects

The principal effects of the Bellow's Breath can be seen in both the physical body and the subtle energy system. On the physical level, residual air from the lungs is purged and toxins are released. Even full yogic breathing does not completely empty the lungs of the last traces of stale air that remain at the end of an exhalation. However, the rapid succession of sharp exhalations in the Bellow's Breath rid the lungs of this residual air and thus succeeds in totally cleaning the lungs. The diaphragm is strengthened since it participates in the Bellow's Breath even though the participation is largely passive. It is not moved by the contraction of its own muscles but is pushed backwards and upwards by the abdomen. Through these movements, the diaphragm is kept mobile and subtle. The student achieves greater control of the abdominal muscles, particularly the large, straight muscles which acquire strength gradually when the exercise is done regularly. The activity of the abdominal muscles tend to eliminate fatty deposits on the abdominal wall. All the organs of the abdominal cavity are toned and massaged as well. This goes for the digestive tract and the glands associated with this region of the physical body. The digestion becomes more active and responsive.

The Bellow's Breath affects the sympathetic nervous system by calming it through hyperoxygenation of the blood and respiratory system. It is a tonic for the entire nervous system.

The Bellow's Breath also changes the oxygen and carbon dioxide balance in the blood. Once you begin the exercise, the carbon dioxide level in the blood falls dramatically. If the exercise is continued for two or three minutes, the whole blood system is cleansed. The normal level is automatically re-established soon after the end of the exercise. The advantage in this exercise is that the temporary drop in the carbon dioxide level in the blood allows the cells to eliminate carbon dioxide and it is replaced with oxygen and a larger dose of Prana than is normal. At the same time as the blood cells lose carbon dioxide they become saturated with oxygen. The resulting increase in cellular activity is particularly important for people who normally lead sedentary lives. In this way, the Bellow's Breath stimulates cellular respiration. Kapalabhati causes all tissues to vibrate. The whole organism trembles under the effect of Kapalabhati, and this vibration has a rejuvenating effect on the entire physical body as well as on the subtle energy system.

CHAPTER XVI

GETTING INTO BALANCE
WITH HARA

Be not wise in thine own eyes; fear the Lord and
depart from evil. It shall be health to thy navel,
and marrow.

—*Proverbs* 2:7-8

Hara

No amount of energy work, breaking energy blockages,
opening and balancing chakras, cleansing auras, etc. will
bring someone into balance if they are unaware of the point
at which their subtle and physical bodies are centered and
balanced. The vast majority of people balance themselves
from a point just above their shoulders and they hang there
like puppets. Their physical body, its posture and the way it
moves, reflects this condition. Because the majority of people are centered just below their head, they tend to experience the world in an inordinately mental way. Moreover,
by being hung from the shoulders like a puppet, people
become prone to many of the problems found in the physical body and the subtle energy system.

Problems such as poor posture, chronic muscle tension
which inhibits the flow of Prana through the subtle energy
system, compressed and twisted spine, cramped body organs

and poor circulation of the blood can be directly linked to being out of balance. Being out of balance puts strain on the joints and ligaments, and it contributes to mental and physical fatigue. Moreover, the process of integration is inhibited when a person is not properly balanced because the second attention, which is a function of the heart and Ajna center, is blocked. Like many of the problems affecting people today, this loss of center, this lack of balance, is a disease of civilization. In less technological times, people related to the world far differently. They were far more integrated with their environment and therefore far more centered. However, in the modern world, the rational mind has become king. By being centered in the shoulders and worshipping rationalism (consciousness), people have lost sight of their true center, their true point of balance. If a person gets caught in the web of thoughts and achievements, forgetting that mind is rooted in the mental body and the mental body is anchored in the I AM, he will lose sight of his true self and will become ensnared in the endless game played by his consciousness and ego. One way for a person to break through the blockages created by an ego trapped in consciousness is by finding his natural center—the center of the physical body as well as the center of the subtle bodies. This center is called *Hara*. It is a person's physical center, but it is more. Hara is an attitude, a way of being, it is the center from which a person moves and acts gracefully, from which a person does what is appropriate at the appropriate time. It is the point of balance from which a person must flow if he hopes to remain centered in the I AM. By being always centered in Hara, a person has access to the energy and consciousness of his subtle bodies which are their birthright.

The Hara, man's center, is located just below the navel; the width of three fingers to be exact. It is from the Japanese that most of our knowledge of Hara comes, and in Japanese the word "Hara" literally means belly. It is in the belly that man finds his equilibrium physically and energetically.

Before we can bring the rest of the physical body into equilibrium and balance, we must become aware and develop Hara. The most efficient way of developing Hara is to begin with an exercise called "Hara Breathing."

Taoist tradition holds that after years of practicing "Hara Breathing" and by activating the Ki energy inherent in Hara, masters were able to melt ice by sitting on it, or they were able to swim in the ocean during winter. You might experiment with the "warming qualities of Hara," called the "Golden Stove," yourself. It can be very practical, especially in winter. If you are out during cold weather and you aren't adequately dressed, try "Hara Breathing" the exercise which follows. You will find it will warm you up immediately.

Hara Breathing

You can practice Hara breathing in any comfortable position as long as your back is straight. It is best not to practice Hara breathing after you have eaten and when you are sleepy. As you progress, you can practice the exercise in a sitting or standing position, but for now I suggest you do it lying down on your back. Begin with your arms at your sides, with your palms up and your fingers loosely extended. Your eyes should be closed and your jaw kept loose by allowing your mouth to drop open comfortably. From this position begin breathing yogically. Breathe yogically for about three to four minutes and then mentally affirm, "I am now deeply relaxed, feeling better than I did before." When you feel ready, bring your mental attention to your Hara, three finger widths directly below your navel. (By paying attention I don't mean concentrate. Concentration as most people understand is a purely mental process in which an individual directs his attention exclusively to one object and closes himself off to everything else.) The preferable technique is to use the second attention.

While you are paying attention, you can allow your conscious mind the freedom to wander where it wishes. After you have focused your second attention on your Hara for just a short time you will feel sensations coming from that vital point. Students often experience warmth, tingling sensations, throbbing sensations, coolness or pressure. None of these feelings should worry you; they are all normal manifestations. After a few moments, in order to activate the Hara further, I want you to place both your hands directly on your Hara. At the same time touch your tongue to your upper palate directly behind your teeth. This will connect the Governor and Conceptual meridians. In this position you are ready to activate your Hara by increasing the level of Prana (Ki) radiating from it and centering your consciousness in it.

To activate Hara, begin by inhaling deeply through the nose into the Hara for a count of five. As you fill Hara with air, visualize that along with the air a fluid is flowing in, filling the Hara with energy and light. This of course is Prana. Retain the breath for a count of five while still focusing your attention on Hara. At this point bring your consciousness to Hara. This will be easiest to do if you imagine yourself feeling and thinking from that point. During the retention you will begin to feel the "Golden Stove" heating up as the level of Prana increases, energizing the organs and tissues of your abdomen.

After you have retained the breath for a count of five, exhale through your mouth for a count of five and bring your tongue back to its normal position. There should be no separation between exhalation and the next inhalation. Only in the retention is the natural rhythm broken. This technique should be done two to three times a week for about 20 minutes. It is an important exercise in psychospiritual integration because by mastering it you return to your true center which is Hara. Karlfried Graf von Durckheim tells us, "The task of gaining the right basic center can be fulfilled only by one who, with perseverance and sincerity, without fear of pain and with great patience overcomes whatever hinders Hara, and furthers that which the developed Hara expresses. To become a complete human being without acquiring the body-soul center is not possible."[1] Being balanced is so important that it is not enough only to bring the breath back to Hara. Everything a person does must be rooted in Hara.

In Japan, Hara is thought of as the point from which the whole person is balanced. Wholeness is a condition which comes when a person finds Hara. Hara can also be thought of not only as a point of balance but as a condition and as a state of balance.

Those with a knowledge of Japanese have found that the concept of Hara has crept into the Japanese language; saying like *Hara No Chiisai Hito*; the man with the little belly or *Hara No Dekite Inai Hito*: the one who has not finished his belly, in Japan are applied to those who are immature or lacking in social grace or the ability to relate well with others and because of their inner discord actually alienate others. On the other hand, actions which spring from the whole man, which are an expression of the I AM are said to come from a man's belly. When a person's thoughts are an expression of the I AM, the Japanese say *Hara De Kangaeru*: to think from the belly or when the sound of a person's voice resonates through his body as an expression of the inner man, the Japanese speak of *Hara Goe*: belly voice.

In my work, I have found that the way a person expresses himself is a reflection of the state of his subtle energy system and of his level of integration. Speaking, posture, movement, thinking: all must be centered in Hara if a person hopes to achieve wholeness. Even the tone of the voice and where it resonates is important. To be an expression of the whole person, it must be centered in Hara at all times. When the voice does not come from Hara, serious difficulties arise because there is a gap between the I AM and the organs of self-expression. When this is the case, the feelings that are expressed come from consciousness, not from the I AM. When deep feelings radiating from the I AM through unconsciousness appear, by being trapped in consciousness the voice may not be available as a vehicle for one's expression. You can see this in people who seem to speak from their neck or head, or who sound hollow or empty when they are angry or upset. The Hara Goe, the voice which comes from Hara, is genuine; it resonates through the whole body. When the voice comes from Hara, it sounds deep and has substance and strength. People unconsciously feel secure around people who speak from Hara. In Japan, if a person's voice doesn't come from Hara, they are considered insincere, untrustworthy and immature.

Overtones

The singing of overtones has the effect of centering the voice in Hara.

For centuries overtones singing was practiced and performed in Tibet, North India, in some Buddhist monasteries in Japan and China. Even some Pygmy tribes in Africa have used overtones. Old folk songs were sung with overtones, and singers in the South-American Andes also practiced overtone singing. Overtones almost always are sung in a religious or spiritual context. Gregorian chants in the late Middle Ages are skillful collections of overtone singing. Eastern musicians and listeners are normally much more conscious of overtones, and they consider the strung tone merely a tool to evolve overtones.

The Tantric tradition kept the knowledge of raising powers and energies through overtone singing a secret up to this century. But now the singing of overtones has again gained importance in Europe after having been almost non-existent for eight centuries.

Today, the singing of overtone offers a person a delightful way to center himself in Hara. A person remembers and recovers lost parts of himself. In this manner he discovers sounds, tones and frequencies of energy he has long ago forgotten. All this has a very comforting and calming effect on a person, allowing him to relax completely and surrender to the I AM, the union of selves.

If you follow the directions in the exercise below, you should have no trouble in successfully singing overtones.

Begin overtone singing by finding a comfortable sitting position with your back straight and begin breathing yogically. Put the tip of your tongue against the top of your mouth while inhaling. Then exhale, while your tongue curls slightly. Let the air out without a sound and with some force but without pressure against your teeth. Your mouth and tongue should be positioned so that there is a small opening between the bottom of your tongue and the roof of your mouth. The tip of your tongue faces backward and the hole allows air to pass through and it is through that space that the overtones are formed.

- Choose a tone that is comfortable for you. It is best when the tone is deep enough to resonate from your Hara.
- It is also important for the sides of your tongue to touch your teeth.
- As you chant, create the sound from your upper palate and nose rather than from your throat.
- When the sound is formed, slide your tongue forward toward your teeth and the overtones will get higher; slide your tongue backwards, and the overtones will get deeper.

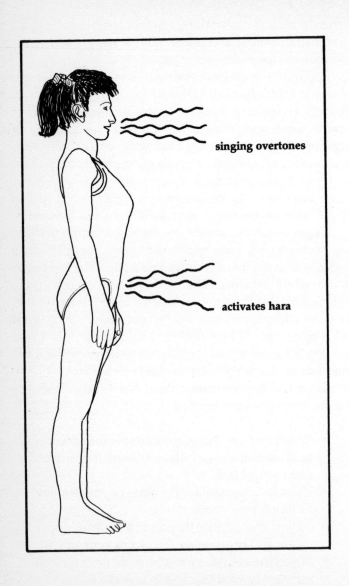

singing overtones

activates hara

Hara can be activated by singing overtones.

- You can also influence the tone by pursing your mouth and adjusting your lips alternatively opening and closing them.

When you sing each vowel (u, o, a, e, i) individually, you will discover that each of them resonates from a different part of your body:

U — in the lower part of the spine
O — in the belly
A — in the heart, chest
E — in the throat
I — in the third eye
Hm — in the crown

I suggest that you practice overtone singing every day for at least ten minutes. Go through each of the vowels so that every part of your body is affected by the vibrations of the overtones. After you are finished chanting, I suggest that you relax for about ten minutes with your eyes closed, breathe yogically and pay attention to how you feel physically, emotionally and mentally. After ten minutes or when you are satisfied, mentally count to yourself from one to five. When you reach the number five, open your eyes. You will feel wide awake, perfectly relaxed and you will be centered in Hara.

Hazrat Inhalat Khan tells us that:

Music is the harmony of the universe . . . it is this harmony that is life manifested in man—who is a miniature of the universe.
That which is most wonderful about music is that through it—without thoughts or concentration—you can get to meditation. Music bridges consciousness with the unconscious, form with formlessness. If there is such a thing that can be realized with the mind but does not have any form—then this is music.[2]

CHAPTER XVII

GENDER IS IN EVERYTHING

In the act of fusion, I know you, I know myself.
I know everybody and I know nothing.

In the Hermetic philosophy we are told "Gender is in everything; everything has its masculine and feminine principles; gender manifests on all planes."[1] The principle of gender and its relationship to health, relationships and spiritual growth is of special importance to us. Gender is manifest on the physical plane as sexuality. Sexuality on the grossest level is the principle which causes male and female to unite for the purpose of procreation. But sexuality must

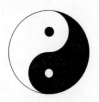

Yin Yang Symbol

be considered as a part of the greater principle of gender which affects and in many ways rules our lives. We can no more define a human being outside one's relationship to gender than we can define a planet without taking into consideration its relationship to the star it revolves around. In the East, gender is represented by this symbol. The symbol represents the polarity, the relationship between masculine (Yang) and feminine (Yin) energy, inherent in everything.

Yin Yang

The Taoist tells us that before the manifest universe came into existence there was nothingness and within the nothingness there was Ching Shing Li: cosmic energy (Prana). At the moment of conception, this cosmic force split into two halves which came to be known by the Chinese

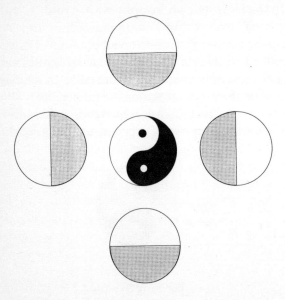

as Yin and Yang. Everything manifest in our universe is defined by its particular balance of Yin and Yang.

Yin represents femininity, body, soul, earth, moon, water, night, cold, darkness, contraction.

Yang on the other hand has opposite characteristics. Yang is masculine, mental, spirit, heaven, sun, day, fire, heat, sunlight, expansion.

Nothing, however, is completely Yin or Yang. Everything has elements of both.

The balance in the universe is the product of the relationship of opposites.

Yin and Yang forces are never static, they constantly change within themselves and in relationship to things outside themselves. An excess of Yin becomes Yang and too much Yang becomes Yin. Water gives us a perfect example of this; water (Yin) by being frozen (Yin) becomes ice (Yang).

Human sexuality cannot be understood outside the concept of Yin/Yang, and cannot be considered as an event separate from other events in the universe. Since events are really only points of interaction between forces (energy fields) with different polarity (concentrations of Yin or Yang), sexuality is a mirror of cosmic relationships.

In the Tantric view, a human being and his/her relationships are a mirror of the universe, or even better, the whole universe in microcosm. The universe itself in the Tantric view is seen as a union of the male and female principle; Yin, the female, is continuously impregnated by the masculine seed (Yang). This continuous creation and the sexual delight aroused by this act are central to Tantric experience and to the Tantric view of wholeness (enlightenment). In Tantra, the universe is continuously being created through the union of opposites. The bliss which results is seen as fundamentally the same as the complete sexual bliss experienced by a couple engaged in sexual union. Thus, in Tantra, human sexuality is elevated beyond the mere act of coitus. It becomes a vehicle for achieving wholeness. In Tantra, it is recognized that through sexual union two individuals can break down the barriers which make them feel separate, and can go beyond separation to the experience of union with each other and union with the universal field.

William Reich recognized this early in this century. He saw that emotional health was related to a person's ability to achieve complete orgasm. Reich stated that in his work he had never come across a neurotic who had the ability to achieve full orgasm. A neurotic, by blocking the complete radiation of his energy, was unable to experience complete orgasm because his fear precluded surrender, the necessary element for free radiation of energy, in this case from the second chakra. Reich saw orgasm as more than simple ejaculation, a function of the sexual organs and a release of energy outwardly through the second chakra. In a purely genital ejaculation, energy is actually wasted because the second chakra draws energy from the nearby chakras, pulling it into the second chakra where it is transmuted into sexual energy. Rather than bringing the partners closer together, this form of orgasm actually has the tendency to push them apart. It does this by preventing energy from radiating outwardly from all seven chakras simultaneously. The normal radiation of the third and fourth chakras are particularly disrupted when this happens. By disrupting the free radiation of energy through the third and fourth chakra, tenderness, love and the normal closeness partners feel for each other is disrupted. Usually, after a purely genital ejaculation, the partners have a desire to quickly part because they feel separate and this causes them pain.

On the other hand, in a healthy orgasm it is the energy of the second chakra which is transmuted. The excitement of the partners increases the energy at the second chakra, and because this increased energy is not stopped by blockages in the energy system or tension in the musculature, it is transmuted into the complete spectrum of human energy, being stepped down to the first chakra and stepped up all the way through the seventh. This increased Prana radiates through the nadis, exciting the entire nervous system. This directly affects the entire body, especially the skin which becomes flushed and more sensitive. The excess energy fills the auras and as the fields intersect, the partners experience total union with one another which is synonymous with complete orgasm. At the moment of climax the seven chakras of each partner explode simultaneously, uniting them on all levels. Because of the full orgasm they experience, not only do they experience more energy but they experience deep intimacy and transcendental love.[2]

In the Symposium, Plato has Hephalstus ask a question which goes to the core of what we all intuitively sense about sexuality. Hephalstus asks: "Is it not perhaps this for which you long, a perfect, mutual fusion so that you will never be sundered from each other by day or night? If this is what you wish, I am ready to melt you and weld you together with fire into one and the same individual so as to reduce you to one single being instead of the two which you were beforehand; in this way you may live united to each other for the whole of your lives ... "[3]

In psychospiritual integration like Tantra, a person calls on energies of the human body which are usually dismissed by more conventional spiritual and psychological schools. Not only don't we dismiss them, we actively cultivate them. The Tantric saint was considered the very antithesis of a spiritual being. "He is so happy" we are told "as to seem crazy; his eyes roll, reddened with wine. He sits on silk cushions surrounded by works of art, eating hot pork cooked with chillies. At the left side sits a girl skilled in the arts of love, with whom he drinks and repeatedly has ecstatic sexual intercourse . . . "[4]

It is not only Tantra which views the release of sexual energy as central to the experience of wholeness. Alice Bailey tells us: "The dense physical externalization of this center (second chakra) is to be found in the gonads, the human organs of generating—viewing them as a basic unity, though temporarily separated in the present dualistic expression of the human being. It must be remembered that this separation fosters a powerful impulse toward fusion, and this urge to blend we call sex. Sex is, in reality, the instinct toward unity; first of all, a physical unity. It is the innate (though much misunderstood) principle of mysticism, which is the name we give to the urge to union with the divine."[6]

Sexual energy and its proper expression and transmutation are central to the work of psychospiritual integration. But the first thing that must be understood is that sexual energy is a form of Prana. It is nothing more than a range of frequencies within the complete spectrum of human energy. It can no more be erased or bent into another shape than we could remove or bend the electrical energy which exists within the physical body into something else.

Enhancing the Flow

The normal flow of sexual energy (except during orgasm) is upward from the second chakra through the sushumna all the way to the seventh chakra at the crown of the head. When this flow is disrupted because of fear and blockages in the subtle energy system, the magic, the excitement, the awe we had as children is lost.*

Disruption of sexual energy as it flows upward through

---

* Sexual energy is a range of energy frequencies which include much that we call creative energy, cheerfulness, brightness. In its more active powerful forms it is the energy which fills a person with the feeling of awe, the feeling that the world is somehow a mysterious and magical place. It cuts through the boring and hum-drum like a knife cuts through butter and it fills a person with childlike "wonder."

the subtle energy system is a common problem. It is the leading cause of depression in society today. Depression begins normally at puberty and is found more often in women than men because society puts more restrictions on how a woman expresses sexual energy. Out of fear or confusion, many women try to prevent sexual energy from radiating through their second chakra because they fear they will attract the wrong kind of attention. Unfortunately, by doing this, women inadvertently block the flow of sexual energy upward.

Men often disrupt the flow in another way by indulging in sex (using it like a drug), in this way allowing their energy to spill out of the second chakra rather than naturally flowing upward.

The Sushumna Meditation

As sexual energy flows up the spine, its frequency is stepped up by each chakra it passes through. The exercise below, which I call the Sushumna Meditation, is designed to enhance this flow and to help you transmute sexual energy into higher frequencies as it flows up your spine.

To begin the Sushumna Meditation, find a comfortable position with your back straight. Close your eyes and begin the yogic breath. Breathe yogically for two or three minutes and then bring your attention to your first chakra at the base of your spine. Immediately bring your breath to your first chakra, and through the second attention begin to feel the feelings associated with the chakra. Keep your attention at the first chakra for about two minutes. From the first chakra, a centimeter at a time, slowly move your attention and your breath up your spine. Feel the energy and feelings of each vertebra until you reach your second chakra which, when stimulated by your mental attention and your breath, will begin to vibrate. At the point of vibration you will feel the feelings associated with the chakra, and for about two minutes feel the energy there in its fullness.

After two minutes, or when you feel satisfied, slowly draw your attention and breath upward along the spine one centimeter at a time until you reach the third chakra. Then experience the energy associated with the third chakra in its fullness for two or three minutes. Continue in this way through the seventh chakra. If there is a lack of sensation, pressure or pain at any point, this indicates that the energy is being blocked. If this is the case, simply spend extra time applying your mental attention and your breath to the area. Don't force or strain yourself in order to feel something. If after a short time there is still a lack of sensation, just move onward. After a few days of practicing the exercise, the flow will improve and blockages will be released. Continue the exercise in the same way until you reach the seventh chakra. After you have finished, relax for about five minutes, breathe yogically and pay attention to how you feel. After five minutes or when you feel satisfied, open your eyes. You will feel wide awake, perfectly relaxed and better than you did before.

Tsing

In the East, a form of sexual energy is called *Tsing*. This energy is produced when a man and woman are together even if they don't make physical contact. It is produced by the tension inherent between Yin and Yang. There are three levels of Tsing, each level being more intense than the one before. The level of Tsing grows in proportion to the levels of Yin and Yang present in the individuals. Where there is an erotic attraction, the couple becomes polarized as the female feels more feminine and the male more masculine. This produces more Tsing, and this form of Prana can alter consciousness and intoxicate the man and woman. An elementary form of Tsing is aroused whenever a man and woman are in contact. Some societies have strict conven-

presence of this elementary form of human magnetism. "This applies to the rule that no woman can visit a man except in the presence of another man, particularly if the first man is married. The rule applies to all women, for sex has no age, and to break the rule even in the most innocent of ways is to have sinned."[6]

A more intense level of Tsing occurs when physical contact is made between a man and woman. This contact can be anything from holding hands to embracing and kissing. The third level of Tsing is reached when intercourse takes place and the partners embrace each other. This third level is the limit of intimacy reached by people who are still unaware of the transcendent nature of sexual energy. To those who view the third Tsing stage as the ultimate experience possible between two people and the most profound experience of sexual contact, there is a deep misunderstanding of the extent of human intimacy.

Through the act of sexual union, two people can actually have the transcendal experience of union with each other and the universal field. Through this experience both partners can experience themselves as whole and totally integrated. That is the reason why the beloved is revered in the East, because through intimate contact with the beloved, union is achieved first with another person and then with the universal field.

Surrender

The first step a person must take in enhancing and improving the flow of sexual energy through the subtle energy system is to free him/herself from the taboos that society has put on its normal and healthy expression. At the roots of humanity's problem with sexuality is the fear of personal extinction, which results from complete sexual union. Sex, by uniting two people energetically and physically and allowing them to melt into union, is inherently threatening to an ego dominated by consciousness.

In true sexual intimacy there is a momentary blotting out of separateness and the experience of separation is replaced by the experience of union. Fear is consciousness' way of preventing this form of union. Fear makes a person contract, and contraction is the antithesis of surrender. The need to surrender is so important in human interaction in general, and sexuality in particular, that it cannot be glossed over lightly.

The ability to surrender to achieve complete sexual union can be likened to death. At the moment of union and orgasmic release, a person transcends the limits imposed upon him/her by the physical body and conscious mind, and with the help of the beloved achieves union and thus transcendence. The Tantric masters before us acknowledged the transcendent nature of sex and used the act of lovemaking as a tool for achieving union with the universal field. Sex became the expression of their transcendent love . . . the full radiation of the I AM on all levels of causation.

This full radiation is only possible when both partners let go of fear and have the trust to radiate freely. Trust comes about when a person has the courage and honesty to be him/herself and feel him/herself "to be in the body at all times." A person in this condition will perceive the world through the second attention, and the mind will be quiet.

All the chakras will be open and the physical body will be completely relaxed. If any of these conditions are not met by one partner or both, complete intimacy will not be achieved because the personal energy fields will be prevented from merging completely. It is particularly important that the chakras are open during sexual intimacy. The blockage of even one chakra is enough to disupt complete union. Moreover, the blockage of one or more chakras by either partner will disrupt the other partner's corresponding chakra and it will disrupt the flow of energy through the nadis. It will weaken the auric fields and disrupt the balance of Yin and Yang energy of both partners. Blockages of one or more chakras is the cause of many of the common sexual problems and dysfunctions which are so prevalent today.

Complete sexual union is so important for relationship, self-esteem and for achieving wholeness that the proper use and radiation of sexual energy during intercourse cannot be left to chance. Incomplete sexual union and the abuse of sexual energy is such a disaster for the subtle energy that I have included a series of exercises developed by Otto Richter, a well-known movement therapist, which will enhance the flow and radiation of sexual energy through your subtle energy system during sex so that you can achieve complete body orgasm and complete union with your partner.

The exercises below form a six-day program. You should do all the exercises each day for six days prior to lovemaking.

Exercise I — Body Part Isolations

Begin "body part isolations" by putting on some relaxing music with a gentle beat. Begin to focus your attention and breathe into your head and neck. Allow the music to permeate the area. Then bring your second attention to the area. Move your head and neck in different ways and let your consciousness fill the area and radiate from it. If you feel resistance to letting go of your head and radiating from there, then you are probably holding on to your thoughts. Keep reminding yourself to *let go* of the "mind" and experience the area through your second attention; then you will be able to move your head freely. Continue to breathe into this area for at least two minutes.

Next move your second attention to your shoulders. Begin breathing in and out from them. Let the music permeate them and then begin moving them. Do they move freely in all directions up, down, forward and back? Are you carrying any burdens there? If so, shake them loose and let go of the heaviness. Then fill your shoulders with your consciousness. Let your consciousness radiate fully from them for at least two minutes. Next bring your second attention to your elbows. Begin breathing into them and bring your consciousness to them. Feel the music permeate them. Feel the feelings and sensations of the joints. Flexibility is the key word here. With this in mind, observe your willingness to be flexible from your elbows.

The rib cage is a place of particular importance. You can't move your ribs without breathing and you can't breathe without moving your ribs. Get in touch with how they work together. Bring your second attention to your rib cage. Breathe into it and fill it with music and your consciousness for two or three minutes. It may help to put your hands on the ribs to understand how they move forward, back, left, right and in circles.

Bring your second attention to your hips (pelvis) and begin breathing from them. Feel the music within this area. Place one hand on your lower abdomen and the other opposite and begin moving your hips. With your hands in this position you will experience the forward and backward, right and left movements of your hips and pelvis. After a few moments, fill the area with your consciousness and let it radiate from there for at least two minutes. If your hips and pelvis are tight, you are probably holding on to and blocking your sexual energy consciously and deliberately. If this is the case, you can stimulate your pelvis further by moving it to the rhythm of the music.

Focus on your spine. Bring your second attention to it. Breathe in and out from it. Begin to undulate it, making movements like a snake. Feel the sexual energy as it radiates from the lower part of your spine and follow it up your back to your neck and head. As it flows upward, feel it radiate from your spine filling your whole body with a warm and vibrant glow. To move spontaneously from your pelvis you must move other parts of the body as well. But even as you do, continue to bring your consciousness from the point in your pelvis where the sexual energy originates and keep it there for two to three minutes.

Next bring your second attention to your knees, breathe in and out from them and feel the music flowing into them. Experiment with different ways of moving them and fill the area with your consciousness for two or three minutes. Repeat this process with your ankles, your feet, toes, arms, wrists, hands and fingers.

After you have isolated your different body parts, one at a time, and you have felt your consciousness radiating through each part, begin putting the parts together. Start isolating, moving and bringing your consciousness through only your toes and feet. Then add your ankles and your knees. From your knees add your hips and so on until your consciousness is radiating simultaneously through each body part. Finally, you will be moving your entire body at the same time. Your energy will be radiating freely from each part and you will be completely in your body. After about five minutes of full body movement, come to a resting position and relax for about five minutes paying attention to how you feel physically, emotionally and mentally.

This exercise integrates the movements, energy and sensations of your physical body and etheric double. It reminds you that your body can move spontaneously and holistically through the integration of its own centers of consciousness.

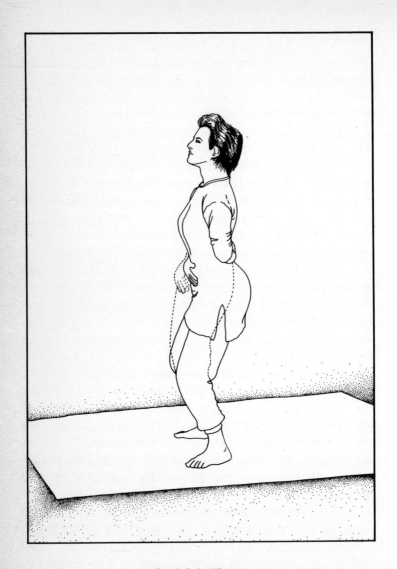

The Pelvic Thrust

Exercise II — The Pelvic Thrust
(to be done with rhythmic music)

Begin the Pelvic Thrust by standing with your feet planted firmly on the floor and knees slightly bent. Then begin moving your pelvis to the music. Pay attention to how your pelvis moves. In particular notice how it can be pushed all the way forward and up and then tilted all the way back as you arch the spine. It will help to put your hands on the front and back of your pelvis for a better point of reference for these movements. Bring your second attention to the area in and around your first and second chakra. Remember, in this area lies the serpent energy, Kundalini. To get both sexual energy and Kundalini flowing properly you will have to take a look at all of your conditioning concerning sex. Old voices from the past will haunt you with thoughts like, "Don't move erotically," "Don't touch yourself there," "It's bad," or "Sex is dirty." The truth of the matter is that sexual energy and Kundalini are the great storehouses of Prana and you must be able to generate and radiate these forms of energy in all situations appropriately.

Once you've been moving from the pelvis for a short time and you are feeling free in that area, bring your arms up over your head in a relaxed position. Then thrust your pelvis forward allowing your spine to begin to undulate. As you tilt your pelvis back, your spine will naturally begin a new undulation. Let sounds accompany each thrust, be sure that they reflect the feeling there and that they resonate through your body. Continue with the movements for at least three minutes and let yourself enjoy them completely.

By doing the Pelvic Thrust you will experience the pelvic region loosening up. Muscles will relax and energy will flow better. After you have completed the exercise, rest in a lying position on your back with your eyes closed for about five minutes and pay attention to how you feel mentally, emotionally and physically.

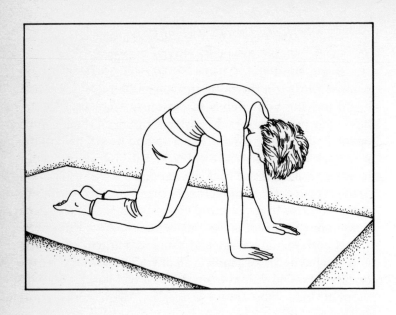

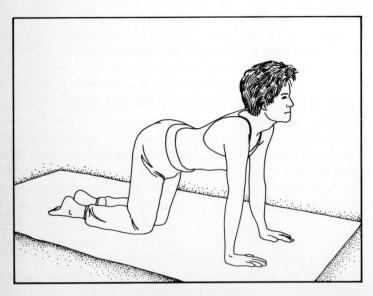

The Running Cat

Exercise III — The Running Cat
(accompanied to rhythmic music)

Begin the Running Cat on your hands and knees. As you breathe in through your nose, arch your spine upward (like an angry cat), tuck your chin all the way to your chest and push your pelvis forward. Both the inhalation and movement should be done very slowly. When you've completed your inhalation without separation between inhalation and exhalation, exhale through your mouth, stick out your tongue as far as you can and arch your spine downward. At the same time, tilt your pelvis back and bring your head up as far as you can without straining. Execute the movement slowly while you exhale. Then repeat both parts four or five more times, or until it becomes second nature and you don't have to think about it.

Begin to quicken the pace. All the movements should be done with the second attention active. Let the movements become as fast as possible and continue them rapidly for at least one minute, or as long as you can without straining. Then gradually slow down the pace until you finally stop. After you stop, lie down on your stomach with your arms at your sides for about five minutes. Breathe yogically and pay attention to how you feel mentally, emotionally and physically. This exercise helps release energy trapped in and around your solar plexus. By releasing energy there you will feel more trusting and connected to your partner. As you connect with your partner from this chakra, you will experience a deep sense of belonging which will facilitate the surrender necessary for achieving complete intimacy and union.

Exercise IV — The Snake Push

To begin the Snake Push, lie down on your back, your knees up and your feet as close to your buttocks as possible. Your feet should be flat on the floor, and your arms at your

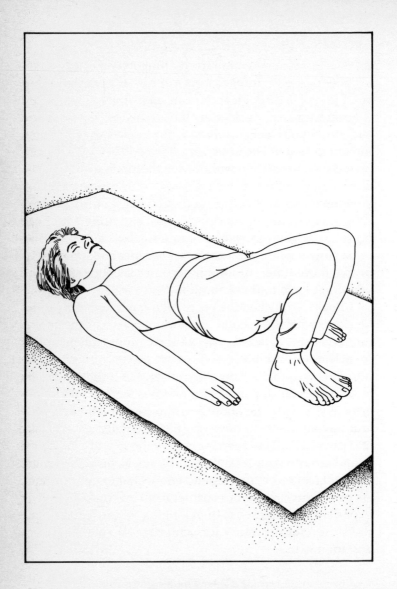

The Snake Push

sides. Begin breathing yogically while you are in this position. In the first movement slowly push your pelvis up, lifting your spine off the floor, vertebra by vertebra. As you lift your pelvis, you will feel the muscles of your thighs and lower abdomen stretch and become more elastic. Make sure the rest of your body is completely relaxed as you stretch the muscles of your legs and abdomen. As you finish the movement, all your weight will be supported by your feet and shoulders and your back will be fully arched. Hold the position for at least one minute if you can, then release the pose very slowly by rolling your spine back onto the floor beginning at the neck and moving down. As you finish, the pelvis will come to a resting position, flat on the floor. Repeat this exercise three times. Then relax for about five minutes lying on your back with your arms at your sides and pay attention to how you feel physically, emotionally and mentally.

The exercise teaches the physical body how to simultaneously integrate feminine and masculine energy. It strengthens the muscles by stretching them, and by helping the muscles become more elastic you will gain a greater degree of control over your movements.

Exercise V — "Yes Mudra"

To begin the "Yes Mudra," lie with your back on the floor, legs together with knees bent up and feet on the floor as close to your buttocks as possible. Your arms should be at your sides with your palms up. Inhale through your nose and on exhalation say "Yes" audibly to yourself. Slowly let your legs fall apart while your feet push against each other. Continue to repeat "Yes" to yourself. You will feel yourself become more open and receptive as you repeat it. At the same time your legs will open wider until your knees are almost touching the floor and the area around your second chakra will relax. After you have relaxed fully in this position, rest in it for about five minutes, then bring your legs up slowly until your knees are back together. Then relax for about five minutes and pay attention to how you feel physically, emotionally and mentally.

Exercise VI — Becoming Honest
These exercises should be done daily, one after another, for six days before lovemaking. On the day of your lovemaking, take some time to just lie down and rest. While you are relaxing, ask yourself the question "Is there anything that I want to tell my partner but have been avoiding?" and, "Am I being honest with myself in this relationship?" These questions are important because your ability to be honest with yourself will determine whether you can be honest with your partner. Without this basic honesty as a foundation, all your communication will be tainted with pretentiousness. Where there is pretentiousness, there is no room for intimacy.

Next I want you to honestly express your innermost feelings about your partner. You should do this after you have completed the first five exercises. This does not necessarily mean to run to the telephone and dump all the anger you've been storing up on your lover. Simply be honest about your thoughts and feelings in the moment, and find a way to express them. You can express them through art, through music, you can write about them through poetry or through a letter (which is never mailed). Another effective way is to imagine your partner sitting in front of you. When you get a mental picture of him/her, speak honestly about how you feel. Of course, you may find it best to speak directly to your partner. Do what is most appropriate for you but make sure that which ever way you decide to express yourself, it is done from the heart and it resonates from deep within you.

After doing this series of exercises every day for six

days you will be ready for tantric lovemaking. The goal of tantric lovemaking, it must be remembered, is transcendental union which is made possible by the complete surrender of both partners. According to the Tantric texts, the best time for lovemaking is from 7 p.m. to midnight. The Tantras advise that lovemaking must never be entered into in total darkness. The room you use should be prepared beforehand; it should be clean, pleasing and airy. A number of symbolic articles should be laid out on an elegant cloth beforehand. These include: two glasses and a pitcher of fresh, cold drinking water, a decanter of wine or any favorite alcoholic beverage, two candles in holders, essence of musk, incense or any good perfume.

Once you are together but before you begin lovemaking, take five minutes to breathe yogically with your eyes closed and then activate the second attention. Transcendental lovemaking requires that both parties experience each other fully. This is only possible when the second attention is active. Then visualize sexual intercourse with your partner in your favorite position—step by step from the first touch through climax. Next pour two small glasses of wine and drink together. After you have drunk together, you are now ready for lovemaking.

Traditionally the man begins by undressing his partner while he stands in front of her.

The males places his fingertips on his partner's body after she is undressed to awaken the dormant forces there. He should touch her heart, the crown of her head, her eyes (a symbolic eye in the center of her forehead) and caress the rest of her body gently.

Then the female partner performs the same procedure on the man. When the woman is finished caressing the man, both partners should lie side by side on the bed, breathing regularly and deeply, joining the rhythms of their breath without touching. Deep relaxed breathing helps to spread the growing excitement to the whole body rather than just the genitals.

A number of positions for coitus are shown in Tantric paintings and sculpture; a favorite has the woman on top. For many people the most comfortable position is on the side. Regardless of what position you use, the important thing is to keep as much contact as possible between the two bodies: eyes locked, faces close enough to inhale each other's breath, hands and fingers interlaced in total communion.

The man should not move or thrust, but just fill the woman with his hard virility as he grasps her buttocks and pushes deep inside her to the root of his sex. The man should feel that he is possessing the woman and is being possessed by her at the same time.

The eyes are the mirror of the soul and it is important that eye contact is maintained. This allows each partner to see the mounting pleasure written on each other's face.

There should be a complete absence of striving and tension. Once the man has entered the woman, all movement should stop. All movement is interior. Lie together like this for perhaps thirty minutes and visualize the flow of energy and love between you. A feeling of heat will rise and be most intense where the genitals meet as if they were being fused together.

If the intimacy is complete at the moment of climax, the muscles of both bodies will contract involuntarily. Searing currents of energy will rhythmically radiate through the body—down the legs to the soles of the feet, through the arms and fingers and through the body from the base of the spine to the top of the head.

The Tantrics describe the blinding moment of union as going beyond the senses, as if there has been an immediate and profound contact with the truth. There is no voice, no image, no vision—only cosmic presence. You cut through the barriers of time and place like a laser. There is no distinction between knower, knowledge and the object of knowledge.

As the energy fields of both partners unite, all boundaries are broken and you feel that you, your partner and the world are all one.

NOTES

Chapter I

1   *The Geeta, The Gospel of the Lord Shri Krishna,* translated by Shri Purchit Swami, Faber and Faber Ltd., London, 1935; p. 44

2   *The Holy Bible, King James Version,* Cambridge University Press, St. Luke 18:19

3   Capra, Fritjof, *The Turning Point,* Fontana Paperbacks, London, 1983; p. 87-88

4   *Ibid.,* p. 88

Chapter II

1   Jacobi, Jolande, *The Psychology of C. G. Jung,* Routledge & Kegan Paul, London, Seventh Edition, reprinted 1975 and 1980; p. 129

Chapter III

1   *The Holy Bible, King James Version,* Cambridge University Press, Isaiah 59:2

2   *Ibid.,* Leviticus 20:24

3   *Ibid.,* The Epistle of Paul to the Galatians 5:16-17

4   *Ibid.,* Luke 10:22

5   Devi, Chitrita, *Upanishads for All,* S. Chand & Co., Ltd., Delhi 1973, Kenopanisad; p. 16

Chapter IV

1   James, William, *The Varieties of Religious Experience,* The Modern Library, New York, 1902, p. 167

2   *Ibid.,* p. 168-169

3   *Ibid.,* p. 169

Chapter V
1   Tagore, Rabindranath, *Gitanjali and Fruit-Gathering*. Bernhard Tauchnitz, 1922, p. 34-35
2   Hesse, Hermann, *Siddharta*, New Directions Publishing Corp., New York, 1957, p. 111

Chapter VI
1   *The Kybalion*, The Yogi Publication Society, Chicago 1912, p. 27
2   Da Free John, *Easy Death*, The Dawn Horse Press, Clearlake, California, 1983; p. 102
3   *The Geeta*, p. 21
4   *Upanishads for All*, Fourth Brahmana (Section 4), p. 337
5   Herrigel, Eugen, *Zen in the Art of Archery*, Vintage Books, New York, 1971, p. 87-89

Chapter VII
1   *Gitanjali and Fruit-Gathering*, p. 47:29
2   Haich, Elisabeth, *Initiation*, Seed Center, Palo Alto, California, 1974, p. 160
3   Janov, Arthur, *The Feeling Child*, Abacus, London, 1982, p. 8
4   *The Kybalion*, p. 35
5   Luce, *Gay Gaer*, Dover Publications Inc., New York, 1971, p. 11
6   *The Feeling Child*, p. 28
7   *Brain Mind Bulletin*, Vol. 8 Nr. 16, Los Angeles, 1983
8   *Ibid.*
9   Jung, C. G., *The Problem of the Attitude Type*, "Essays on Analytical Psychology CW7 par 78"—Collected Works
10 *Holy Bible*, Mark 10:14
11 *Ibid.*, Matthew 21:33-38

Chapter VIII
1   Langenscheidt, *New Pocket Dictionary*, Berlin, 1970; p. 515

2   Rousseau, Jean Jacques, *The Social Contract*
3   Fontain, Jean de la, *Le Cheval s'etant voulu venger du cerf*
4   Rochefoucauld, Francois, Duc de la, *Reflexions*
5   Tao Te King, *Lao Tsu*, Penguin Books, Middlesex, 1963, 48, p. 108
6   Shah, Idries, *A Veiled Gazelle*, The Octagon Press, London, 1978; p. 25
7   *The Kybalion*, p. 32
8   Tillich, Paul, *The Courage to Be*, Yale University Press, New York, 1979, p. 27
9   *Ibid.*, p. 23
10 *Ibid.*, p. 30
11 Merton, Thomas, *The New Man*, Farrar, Straus & Giroux, New York, 1978, p. 90

Chapter IX

1   *Easy Death*, p. 111-112
2   Yogi, Ramacharaka, *Science of Breath*, Yogi Publication Society, Chicago, 104; p. 10

Chapter X

1   *The Kybalion*, p. 39ff
2   *Holy Bible*, The First Epistle of Paul the Apostle to the Corinthians, 3:16
3   Kulvinskas, Viktoras, *Survival into the 21st Century*, 21st Century Publications, Woodstock, 1975; p. 129 and 132
4   Suzuki, D. T., *The Zen Doctrine of No Mind*, Rider Pocket Edition, Reading, Britain, 1983, p. 72
5   *Upanishads for All*, Fourth Chapter, Svetasvata-ropnisad, Section 17, p. 109
6   Bailey, Alice A., *The Soul and Its Mechanism*, Lucis Publishing Company, New York, 1981, p. 43

Chapter XI

1 Ramakrishna, Sri, *Teachings of Sri Ramakrishna*, published by Swami Budhananda, Advaita Eshrama, Calcutta 1975, p. 11

2 *Upanishads for All*, p. 89

Chapter XII

1 Motoyama, Hiroshi, *Theories of the Chakras*, The Theosophical Publishing House, Wheaton, 1981, p. 23

2 *The Soul and Its Mechanism*, p. 119

3 Leadbeater, C. W., *The Chakras*, The Theosophical Publishing House, Wheaton, 1977, p. 72-3

4 *Holy Bible*, John 10:16

5 Lawrence, Brother, *The Practice of the Presence of God*, The Peter Pauper Press, Mount Vernon, 1963, p. 32-3

6 *The Soul and Its Mechanism*, p. 111

7 *The Chakras*, p. 13

8 *Holy Bible*, II Timothy 1:7

9 *Siddharta, A New Direction Book*, p. 107

10 *Upanishads for All*, Svetasvararopanisad 12, p. 91

11 *The Zen Doctrine of No Mind*, p. 97

12 Tao Te Ching, *Lao Tsu*, Penguin Books Ltd., Harmondsworth, 1979, p. 72

13 Sherwood, Keith, *The Art of Spiritual Healing*, Llewellyn Publications, St. Paul, 1985, p. 62

14 Capra, Fritjof, *The Tao of Physics*, Bantam New Age Books, New York, 1980, p. 112

Chapter XIV

1 *Omni* Publication International Ltd., B. Guccione (Editor), New York, Oct. 82, p. 79

Chapter XV

1 Teeguarden, Joma Tarsaa, *Acupressure Way of Health*, Japan Publications Inc., 1978, p. 59

2   Iyengar, B. K. S., *Light on Pranayama*, Unwin Paper-
    backs, London, 1981

Chapter XVI
1   Durckheim, Karlfried Graf von, Mandala Books, London,
    1984, p. 33
2   Hazrat, Inhalat Khan, *Music is the Harmony*, zitiert aus
    Esotera, Obertone

Chapter XVII
1   *The Kybalion*, p. 39
2   Evola, Julius, *The Metaphysics of Sex*, East West Publi-
    cations, London, 1969, p. 43
3   Plato
4   Rawson, Philip, *Tantra*, Thames and Hudson, London,
    1973, p. 9
5   Bailey, Alice, *A Compilation on Sex*, Lucis Press Ltd., Lon-
    don, 1980.
6   *The Metaphysics of Sex*, p. 23

INDEX

On the following pages you will find listed, with their current prices, some of the books now available on related subjects. Your book dealer stocks most of these and will stock new titles in the Llewellyn series as they become available. We urge your patronage.

TO GET A FREE CATALOG

To obtain our full catalog, you are invited to write (see address below) for our bi-monthly news magazine/catalog, *Llewellyn's New Worlds of Mind and Spirit.* A sample copy is free, and it will continue coming to you at no cost as long as you are an active mail customer. Or you may subscribe for just $10 in the United States and Canada ($20 overseas, first class mail). Many bookstores also have *New Worlds* available to their customers. Ask for it.

TO ORDER BOOKS AND TAPES

If your book store does not carry the titles described on the following pages, you may order them directly from Llewellyn by sending the full price in U.S. funds, plus postage and handling (see below).

Credit card orders: VISA, MasterCard, American Express are accepted. Call toll-free within the USA and Canada at 1-800-THE-MOON.

Special Group Discount: Because there is a great deal of interest in group discussion and study of the subject matter of this book, we offer a 20% quantity discount to group leaders or agents. Our Special Quantity Price for a minimum order of five copies of *Chakra Therapy* is $39.80 cash-with-order. Include postage and handling charges noted below.

Postage and Handling: Include $4 postage and handling for orders $15 and under; $5 for orders *over* $15. There are no postage and handling charges for orders over $100. Postage and handling rates are subject to change. We ship UPS whenever possible within the continental United States; delivery is guaranteed. Please provide your street address as UPS does not deliver to P.O. boxes. Orders shipped to Alaska, Hawaii, Canada, Mexico and Puerto Rico will be sent via first class mail. Allow 4-6 weeks for delivery. **International orders:** Airmail – add retail price of each book and $5 for each non-book item (audiotapes, etc.); Surface mail – add $1 per item.

Minnesota residents add 7% sales tax.

Mail orders to:
Llewellyn Worldwide
P.O. Box 64383-721, St. Paul, MN 55164-0383, U.S.A.

For customer service, call (612) 291-1970.
Prices subject to change without notice.

WHEELS OF LIFE
A User's Guide to the Chakra System
by Anodea Judith
An instruction manual for owning and operating the inner gears that run the machinery of our lives. This fully illustrated book will take the reader on a journey through aspects of consciousness, from the bodily instincts of survival to the processing of deep thoughts.

Discover this ancient metaphysical system under the new light of Western metaphors: quantum physics, elemental magick, Kabbalah, physical exercises, poetic meditations, and visionary art. Learn how to open these centers in yourself, and see how the chakras shed light on the present world crises we face today. The modern picture of the Chakras was introduced to the West largely in the context of Hatha and Kundalini Yoga and through the Theosophical writings of Leadbeater and Besant. But the Chakra system is equally innate to Western Magick: all psychic development, spiritual growth, and practical attainment is dependent upon the opening of the Chakras!
0-87542-320-5, 544 pgs., 6 x 9, illus., softcover   **$17.95**

THE ART OF SPIRITUAL HEALING
by Keith Sherwood
Each of you has the potential to be a healer; to heal yourself and to become a channel for healing others. Healing energy is always flowing through you. Learn how to recognize and tap this incredible energy source. You do not need to be a victim of disease or poor health. Rid yourself of negativity and become a channel for positive healing.

Become acquainted with your three auras and learn how to recognize problems and heal them. Special techniques make this book a "breakthrough" to healing power, but you are also given a concise, easy-to-follow regimen of good health to follow in order to maintain a superior state of being. This is a practical guide to healing.
0-87542-720-0, 224 pgs., 5 ¼ x 8, illus., softcover   **$7.95**